Medicare: The Politics of Federal Hospital Insurance

Medicare: The Politics of Federal Hospital Insurance

Judith M. Feder

Lexington Books
D. C. Heath and Company
Lexington, Massachusetts
Toronto

Library of Congress Cataloging in Publication Data

Feder, Judith Morris.
    Medicare : the politics of federal hospital insurance.

    Bibliography: p.
    Includes index.
    1. Hospitals—United States—Finance. 2. Hospital care—United
States—Quality control. 3. Medicare. 4. Insurance, Hospitalization—
United States. 5. United States. Social Security Administration. I. Title.
RA981.A2F4   362.1'1   77–4611
ISBN 0–669–01447–8

Published simultaneously in Canada

Printed in the United States of America

International Standard Book Number: 0–669–01447–8

Library of Congress Catalog Card Number: 77–4611

Contents

Preface

In March 1977, Secretary of Health, Education, and Welfare Joseph Califano announced a major departmental reorganization. Its purpose was to unify administration of the federal government's two major health financing programs—Medicare and Medicaid—which had been run independently, and often without coordination, since their inception. Responsibility for Medicare was removed from the Social Security Administration (SSA), for Medicaid from the Social Rehabilitation Service, and a new agency—the Health Care Financing Administration—was created to administer both programs.

The Carter administration has emphasized the importance of this reorganization for efficient program management, particularly control of fraud and abuse. Of equal or greater importance may be the impact of reorganization on the health policy promoted by the two financing programs. This book, written just before the change was announced, concludes that reorganization was essential to shift Medicare's focus from social insurance to health policy. The book's fundamental premise is that Medicare policy toward hospitals has been profoundly influenced by the perspectives and goals its administrators acquired in a social insurance agency. The social insurance perspective emphasized efficient claims payment rather than controlling the impact of payment on the costs and quality of medical care. Initially reinforced by concern that exercising control would antagonize the hospitals and threaten Medicare's survival, this perspective became entrenched over time as administrators grew accustomed to operating procedures and working relationships with the hospitals. Despite internal skepticism about the appropriateness of some established arrangements, SSA sought to avoid the administrative disruption and political conflict associated with change. Even when external pressure for change arose, SSA's response was cautious and limited. As a result, Medicare has continued to support inadequate and unsafe hospitals and to exacerbate hospital cost inflation.

The transfer of authority over Medicare to a new agency could alter administrative commitments and perspectives. Under the Health Care Financing Administration, Medicare is a major part of a new agency's responsibility for health financing, instead of a small part of SSA's responsibility for social insurance. If reinforced by changes in personnel, lines of authority, and leadership, this transfer could mean a new conception of the ends and means of hospital payment under Medicare.

This change will depend on both a conscious administrative effort and external support for an alternative approach to policy. As this book will show, SSA's behavior has been influenced as much by a rational assessment of its political environment as by its administrative predispositions. Over the last decade, pressure from the Congress and the executive branch for payment policies that encourage the efficient delivery of medical care has been intermittent and limited. Without more pressure in this direction, reorganization alone is unlikely to alter policy.

Although it is too early to predict what the reorganization's impact on Medicare policy will be, now is the time to decide what the impact should be and to take measures to achieve it. These decisions require an understanding of the last decade of Medicare administration and the factors that have shaped it. The following account of Medicare's implementation will provide that understanding.

Acknowledgments

I began this study at The Brookings Institution, continued it with a grant from the Social Security Administration at the Policy Center, Inc.,[a] and completed it at the National Center for Health Services Research. My affiliation with these organizations and Harvard University provided both the financial support and professional stimulation that made this book possible.

Among the many individuals from whose assistance I benefited, I am particularly indebted to the present and former Medicare officials who were willing to share their experience; to Robert Gallucci, Judith May, Diane Rowland, and Peter Schuck for advice and moral support; to Patrick O'Donoghue, Rick Carlson, Karen Davis, Clark Havighurst, Ted Marmor, Roger Noll, Ronald Vogel, and the staff of the Policy Center, Inc., for their participation in the SSA-funded project; to Gerald Rosenthal, Norman Weissman, Gail Lasdon, Mary Lee, Gary Shannon, Sharon Soroko, Daniel Walden, and William Weissert for their encouragement and support at the National Center; to Professors Barrington Moore, Jr. and James Q. Wilson for invaluable instruction along the way to a Ph.D.; to typists Madge Johnston, Shirley Minasi, Charlotte Mullinix, and Teresa Spaid for patience and perseverance; and to my husband Stanley and my son Sam, for confidence and perspective when I needed them most.

[a]The final report for this grant (No. 10-P-57693/8-01), on which this book is based, was published as *The Character and Implications of SSA's Administration of Medicare* (Denver: Spectrum Research, Inc., 1975).

Medicare: The Politics of Federal Hospital Insurance

1

Alternative Strategies for Medicare's Implementation

In 1935, the designers of social security considered including national health insurance in their legislation. But fearing physician opposition that could jeopardize their whole program, they decided to leave it out. The same men then spent much of the next thirty years trying to put it back in. Medicare was the result. Its provisions reflected two major compromises believed necessary for its enactment. First, Medicare did not cover the whole population, but provided health insurance only to the elderly. Strategists believed that the appeal of helping the elderly would overcome physician opposition to any federal health insurance. Second, the Medicare law explicitly promised that the federal insurance program would not interfere in the practice of medicine or the structure of the medical care industry.

At the same time, the authors of the law recognized that paying for medical care for twenty million people would mean an enormous influx of dollars into the health care system. How that money would be spent had major implications for taxpayers and the health care industry. Despite its promise of noninterference, the law therefore required program administrators to establish conditions for payment—a requirement that inevitably would lead to some interference. Fulfilling these conflicting obligations became the task of the Social Security Administration (SSA), the agency from which key Medicare strategists had come.

The potential impact of just one part of the Medicare program, payment to hospitals, on the size and costs of the hospital industry was considerable. The elderly comprise approximately one-quarter of the average hospital's patients. Before Medicare, much of the care they obtained had been provided as charity. Medicare ended this situation, providing a substantial potential for increased hospital revenues. Because most hospitals are nonprofit institutions, any surplus of revenues over expenditures does not go to stockholders. Instead it goes back into the hospital in salaries, services, and facility expansion. Furthermore, when a hospital uses its "profit" or net income to expand its services, its operating costs increase. Patients or insurance programs are then asked to pay these additional costs. If the hospital again earns a "profit," it expands further, and costs even more the following year. The Medicare program, enacted to pay for hospital care for the elderly, thus offered potential support for the almost unlimited growth of each hospital used by the elderly.

Faced with this possibility, Medicare administrators had to make several choices as they developed a policy on hospital payment. This is a study of the

1

choices they made. The first decision was whether to pay for care in any hospital the elderly used. At the time of enactment, many hospitals were inadequately staffed, poorly equipped, and fundamentally unsafe. Their contribution to patient care was questionable. Congress therefore specified that Medicare not support substandard care and included in the law some basic requirements for adequacy of care. The law further authorized the secretary of health, education, and welfare to establish additional requirements as necessary to protect the health and safety of Medicare beneficiaries. In implementing this authority, SSA had to decide what to require of a hospital's performance or quality before finding it eligible for Medicare funds. They had to choose between perpetuating inadequate hospitals with Medicare funds or denying them participation, potentially forcing their improvement or disappearance.

Among its specific quality requirements, the law included one intended to control the costly expansion of services that Medicare might produce. The law required that each hospital establish a "utilization review committee" of the hospital's physicians and other personnel, to review and evaluate the care they gave. Through this review process, its advocates believed, physicians would keep each other from offering unnecessary services.

Although members of the medical profession were among advocates of utilization review, it was a new concept in 1965 and few committees actually existed. Including it as a requirement for hospital participation made Medicare administrators directly responsible for the establishment of a new professional practice. Along with development of health and safety requirements, implementation of this provision required a choice—to evaluate or ignore how physicians and hospitals practiced medicine.

Determining the method of hospital payment also entailed a decision on the extent of government control. Inflation in hospital costs is greater if each hospital has complete autonomy in pricing its services. If buyers pay whatever hospitals ask, costs spiral. In fact, this is a fairly accurate description of what has occurred with the spread of health insurance. As consumers have become less responsible for payment of their medical bills, market constraints on hospital charges have declined. Insurers have failed to develop alternative constraints. Medicare administrators had to choose whether to follow that pattern or develop controls of their own.

To overcome industry opposition, Medicare strategists patterned the law's payment provisions on principles developed by the hospitals and their long affiliated insurance operation, Blue Cross. Instead of specifying payment of charges for services rendered, these principles called for payment by the insurer of a hospital's *costs*. Agreement on this approach did not produce uniformity in the private sector, however, for costs can be defined in a variety of ways. Cost reimbursement, as it is called, requires decisions on the measurement of costs and the specific costs to be included in payment for patient care. It is necessary, for example, to decide how much, if anything, an insurer should pay for nurses' training, medical research, facility construction, etc., and what share of these costs are attributable to its beneficiaries. These decisions were made in numerous ways in the private sector, and their impact on hospital revenues varied considerably. In choosing whether to be stringent or liberal in measuring costs, SSA had to define Medicare's responsibility for financing the hospital and medical industry.

Along with deciding what kind of services would be paid for and how costs would be measured, SSA had to decide whether there would be any upper limit set on costs. This decision applied to specific items like administrative salaries and to a hospital's relative efficiency overall. When these problems arose in legislative deliberations, Medicare strategists adopted the position of the hospital trade association, the American Hospital Association (AHA). A hospital's incurred costs should be paid, said the AHA, unless they were "out of line" with those of other similar hospitals. This intent was specifically included in the legislative history, along with instructions to pay only "reasonable costs." Responsible for turning such generalities into specifics, administrators were left to choose whether and how to evaluate the legitimacy of a particular hospital's costs and what to do if they found them unsatisfactory.

In sum SSA faced choices in the areas of hospital quality—eligibility and utilization review—and hospital financing. Theoretically, SSA could have handled each of these choices independently, reacted to events, and simply "muddled through" the issues in hospital payment. I will argue, however, that SSA's policy choices reflected a consistent strategy toward program implementation.

That strategy could have taken two fundamentally different forms. The first would have been to base policy choices on a conscious assessment of political pressure. This *balancing strategy* is consistent with a pluralist theory of politics and a related theory of bureaucracy. According to Truman[1] and others, a bureaucracy seeking survival will make policy reflect the influence of competing pressure groups. This does not necessarily mean that the bureaucracy lacks policy goals of its own; but with a balancing strategy, the bureaucracy seeks to identify relevant political actors, weighs their capacity to aid or threaten program survival, and selects the policy that minimizes political conflict.

The alternative strategy would be to base choices on a calculation of how to finance hospital care most effectively and efficiently. The *cost-effectiveness strategy* is consistent with Weber's view of bureaucracies as efficiently pursuing their stated objectives. With this theory, the bureaucracy assesses the impact of hospital payment on cost and quality, and selects a course that achieves maximum health care value per dollar spent. Although this bureaucracy does not ignore its political environment, it is willing to risk political conflict to achieve its objectives.

Each strategy presents a different set of answers to SSA's policy choices. The balancer's answers would come from pressures in the political environment.

On both quality and costs, SSA could expect to face considerable pressure from the hospitals, seeking maximum funds and minimum control. If hospitals were the only active pressure group in SSA's environment, policy would reflect their interests. But this was not the case. In the quality area the Public Health Service (PHS)—the health professionals in the Department of Health, Education, and Welfare (HEW)—and other public health professionals saw Medicare as an opportunity to upgrade hospital quality, and therefore advocated stringent minimum standards of hospital eligibility and government oversight of medical practice. Facing these competing pressures, a balancing agency would weigh their relative influence on program survival and base its policy on the appropriate compromise.

On costs, the hospitals' interests in maximum reimbursement would also encounter opposition. Uncontrolled payments to hospitals would mean increased taxes or inability to finance other federal programs. Thus Congress and the president, both of whom have other program interests and prefer to avoid raising taxes, have a stake in cost control. A balancing strategy would take these interests as well as the hospitals' into account, continually compromising hospital demands with congressional and executive concern with the budget.

The agency pursuing a cost-effectiveness strategy would arrive at its policy choices in a totally different way. Rather than weigh interests and influence in the political environment, it would make a "technical" assessment of the resources available and the most efficient and effective way to employ them. This would entail establishing both quality and cost objectives and imposing conditions on payment to achieve them. The cost-effectiveness strategist would determine minimal quality criteria and pay for services only in hospitals able to meet them. Exceptions would be made only where no hospitals in an area could qualify, and policy would be designed to improve conditions in these hospitals. Similarly, objectives would be defined for utilization review, procedures for its implementation developed, compliance required, and performance evaluated.

On payment, the cost-effectiveness strategist would evaluate the impact of reimbursement policies on the hospital system—noting that paying each hospital's costs at whatever level the hospital chose would encourage duplication of services, unnecessary hospital beds, consumption of unnecessary or excessive services, and open-ended costs. The cost-effectiveness strategist would design reimbursement policies to avoid this occurrence. This could be done in two ways.

First, administrators could take seriously the industry's and the law's exception to payment of costs that were "out of line" or "unreasonable," and establish cost constraint by regulation. Reimbursement policies would therefore include comparisons among hospitals, specification of efficient delivery of services, and the imposition of "reasonable" cost ceilings.

Alternatively, or in addition, administrators could shape reimbursement to encourage market constraints on hospital costs. Although the most powerful market constraints might come from having consumers pay a significant portion of their medical expenses, this approach was limited by the law's specifications for consumer cost-sharing. Medicare payment policy could, however, affect the supply side of the medical market. Specifically, reimbursement policy could encourage the growth and development of organized medical systems delivering comprehensive services more efficiently, that is, at lower total costs, than providers in general. The primary example is the prepaid group practice or health maintenance organization, whose members receive comprehensive care in return for payment made in advance. In contrast to the fee-for-service system, where hospital and physician incomes rise with the number of services they provide, the prepaid system, with its income set in advance, has incentives to minimize the costs of care. Members of these organizations tend to use the hospital far less than consumers in general, thereby reducing the costs of care. Although the incentives of prepaid group practice raise concerns about quality control, administrators interested in cost-effective delivery would certainly explore its potential.

Beyond these particular choices, one would expect the cost-effectiveness strategist to evaluate payment policies continually for their impact on costs and quality. If the law proved an obstacle to what administrators considered desirable changes, as with cost-sharing, for example, we would expect them to seek legislative amendment.

This study will identify the strategy actually followed by SSA for dealing with hospitals over the last ten years in four areas—hospital eligibility, utilization review, reimbursement, and cost control. The purpose of the study is to explain why SSA followed this strategy rather than the alternative. This analysis of what SSA did and why will give us new insights on how a bureaucracy deals with discretionary authority, political pressure, and economic and professional interests in American society.

Note

1. David B. Truman, *The Governmental Process: Political Interests and Public Opinion* (New York: Alfred A. Knopf, 1964), especially chapter 14.

2

Hospital Quality: The Development and Implementation of Conditions for Participation

When Congress enacted Medicare, it decided to accompany the promise to pay for hospital care with some assurance of its quality.[1] The law therefore specified minimal quality standards that hospitals would have to meet to get paid and authorized the secretary of HEW to develop other requirements "as necessary in the interest of health and safety."[2] Authors of the law did not intend this authority to usurp the health industry's own quality control activity. On the contrary, Congress explained:

The inclusion of these conditions is designed to support the efforts of the various professional accrediting organizations sponsored by the medical and hospital associations, health insurance plans, and other interested parties to improve the quality of care in hospitals.[3]

Government strategist Wilbur Cohen underscored this intent with legislative provisions that declared all hospitals accredited by the industry's own Joint Commission on Accreditation of Hospitals (JCAH)[4] automatically in compliance with Medicare quality requirements and prohibited the secretary from imposing any requirements more stringent than the commission's.[5] These provisions left the secretary and SSA to establish quality standards for hospitals that did not have the industry's own stamp of approval.

This stamp originated in the medical profession's drive to establish standards for medical education.[6] In developing criteria for professional training, the American College of Surgeons found it impossible to separate "the training of a surgeon in a hospital from the operation of that hospital."[7] Their standards and those of the joint commission therefore became the industry's definition of the structural, organizational, personnel, and service requirements for acceptable hospital care. More specifically, accreditation criteria are:

basic definitions of (1) the kinds of services that should be available in a given type of health care facility or program; (2) the kinds of professional personnel who should be there to provide the services, including qualifications and adequate numbers relative to patient loads; (3) the way in which the personnel should be organized to provide the services and maintain the quality control, e.g., medical staff committees, by-laws, etc.; (4) the kinds of policies and administrative organizations and procedures that should be present; (5) the kinds of equipment and physical facilities required, together with definitions of adequacy for safety, cleanliness, and sanitation; and (6) other areas of importance to health and safety, such as dietary service, drugs, and medical records.[8]

Theoretically, these definitions assure the consumer who seeks hospitalization that an institution called a hospital can provide diagnosis, treatment, and care consistent with prevailing professional practice. If, for example, someone is rushed to a "hospital," standards are intended to assure him that the institution is organized and equipped to respond to him quickly, to diagnose his condition, and to treat and care for him as his condition requires in a sanitary and safe environment. In purchasing medical care, where consumers are frequently unable to choose or evaluate the care they receive or to correct a mistake once made,[9] this assurance can provide valuable protection.

It is not, however, a guarantee of quality care. Setters of standards emphasize that they are looking only at a hospital's capacity to perform, not the performance itself.[10] Other ways to assess quality focus on the activities of health professionals in managing patients, or the "process" of delivering care, and on the "outcomes" or results of care for patient health and satisfaction. The relationship among these measures of care has not been clearly established. Professionals assume that "appropriate structure increases the probability of good care, which, in turn, improves the likelihood of favorable outcomes."[11] A few studies have tested this assumption, with somewhat mixed results.[12] Hence, the impact of "structural" standards is subject to question.

In addition, consumers and health professionals have questioned whether JCAH standards have been adequately enforced. There is substantial evidence that accreditation is a political process, in which failure to meet standards frequently does not result in denial of accreditation.[13]

Despite these qualifications on the value of structural standards, failure to meet them sometimes has obvious consequences for patient care. Because of its inadequacies, D.C. General Hospital was granted only one year provisional accreditation in 1970. Patient groups and medical staff, who felt that JCAH should have denied the hospital accreditation altogether, complained of drug shortages, lack of nurses, lost and incorrect medical records, inaccurate and unavailable lab reports, lost X-rays, and other deficiences amounting to approximately seventy-six violations of more than sixteen JCAH standards.[14]

The house staff reported:

In a recent sampling of 55 requests for patient records made to the medical records department, only one out of six could be retrieved. In another sampling 15 out of 30 were missing. Because past records often cannot be found, the medical staff is unable to properly plan future care, communicate with other physicians and professionals contributing to the patient's care, or provide data for use in research and education.[15]

In 1975 D.C. General did lose its accreditation. At that time, there were complaints of structural deficiencies, inadequate record-keeping, and equipment breakdowns that endangered patients' lives.[16]

Similar problems have arisen in numerous public hospitals across the country.[17] The JCAH denied accreditation to Boston City Hospital with the following observations:

The attention of the medical staff and administration is directed to the major deficiencies which include failure to properly maintain existing automatic sprinkler systems; lack of automatic fire extinguishing systems . . . delay in completion of medical records; lack of a sufficient number of graduate registered nurses for full patient coverage; need for additional qualified therapeutic dietitians; need to revise medical staff by-laws; need for relocation of surgeon's dressing room to reduce potential of outside contamination; need for architectural segregation of the labor delivery room and newborn nursery and urgent need for adequate facilities to allow for proper separation of infected gynecological patients from the obstetrical-newborn area.[18]

Public hospitals, whose clientele often cannot afford to pay for medical care, have been less likely to be accredited than have private nonprofit hospitals, but they are not the only hospitals that have not met professional standards. As of the early sixties, JCAH accreditation was associated with both the form of hospital ownership and hospital size.[19] Hospitals operated for profit were least likely to be accredited, and were criticized for using untrained, unsupervised staff, resulting in mistreatment of patients.[20] As for hospital size, until 1967 the JCAH did not generally survey hospitals with fewer than twenty-five beds.[21] When they changed their policy, very few small hospitals were accredited.[22] In 1965, SSA estimated that nonaccredited hospitals comprised 40.2 percent of nonfederal short-term general hospitals (approximately 2,700 hospitals) but only 13.4 percent of the beds—in other words, a large number of small hospitals were not accredited.[23]

Some of these hospitals were unclean and unsafe, like those described above. Many of them lacked adequate staff.[24] Their biggest accreditation problem, however, seems to have been their overall failure to measure up to contemporary standards of technology, staffing and medical practice. Feather Hair, in her study of accreditation, characterized their situation:

Small, rural and poor communities tend to have small, understaffed hospitals unable to afford the expanding number of new machines and technologies developed by modern medical science.[25]

In 1965 care in nonaccredited hospitals simply fell short of the level that most of the nation's hospital care had reached.[26]

What to do about these hospitals was a problem for Medicare administrators. If they made no requirements of nonaccredited hospitals, beneficiaries would have no assurance that the hospitals they used were capable of providing the care they required and could obtain elsewhere.[27] If on the other hand

Medicare imposed higher standards on hospitals than they were able to meet, there would be other difficulties. Elderly patients accustomed to using those hospitals would have to go elsewhere. Unless alternative facilities were readily available, this would deny them the benefits Medicare was supposed to provide. Hospitals denied certification would lose a major source of patient revenue, forcing many of them out of business. Thus Medicare administrators had to make a choice: impose professionally acceptable quality standards and deny certification to large numbers of hospitals, or ignore their responsibility for quality and certify hospitals regardless of their relative and absolute inadequacies.

This chapter will show that SSA made its choice by focusing on what would make the program politically successful. Medicare officials weighed the political costs and benefits of alternative courses of action in terms of the responses of beneficiaries, hospitals, health professionals, and the public at large. Officials believed that Medicare would be most successful if they treated it as an extension of Social Security benefits and avoided quality enforcement. But they could not attract support for this approach from health professionals who believed that Medicare should upgrade the quality of the nation's hospitals. Because achieving consensus was as important to SSA as other objectives, they compromised, combining professionally acceptable standards with explicitly lenient measures of compliance.[28] Both the process and content of SSA's "educational" approach to hospital certification reflect a balancing strategy.

Policy Objectives

To assure physicians and hospitals that decisions related to the practice of medicine would be made by health professionals, Medicare strategists promised the Congress that SSA would consult the Public Health Service (PHS) in developing quality standards.[29] Consistent with this promise, in the early sixties HEW and SSA officials encouraged PHS to begin work in· this area. Although Surgeons General had for some time avoided National Health Insurance and Medicare as too controversial, PHS activity increased with the likelihood of the program's enactment. The Surgeon General established a unit to work on potential Medicare requirements and staffed it with new personnel interested in quality regulation. In the spring of 1965, when Medicare's passage was virtually certain, SSA requested PHS to develop standards for hospital and other institutional participation in Medicare, and joint SSA–PHS work groups were established.[30]

The PHS officials who undertook this job saw Medicare as a "real opportunity . . . for raising the quality of care provided throughout the country . . . ."[31] By authorizing national standards of quality and financing reviews of hospital compliance, the PHS staff thought that Medicare could upgrade the quality of the nation's hospitals. They approached the development of standards with this objective in mind. At the same time, they noted the problems that hospitals would have in achieving the desired capabilities. They adopted as a model the JCAH's structural accreditation standards, which were acceptable to the industry and represented an absolute minimum level of hospital quality in the eyes of PHS professionals. Furthermore, PHS proposed to distinguish "basic" from "desirable" conditions and to require only the former. They believed that a hospital unable to meet even these should be certified only where no other hospital was available to beneficiaries.[32]

Social Security officials did not challenge PHS definitions of quality but disagreed strongly with the priority they assigned them in Medicare implementation. As far as Medicare administrators were concerned, PHS officials were aiming toward the "millenium" in their stance on quality regulation. The goal of Medicare's architects and chief administrators was far more immediate—to get the program smoothly under way by July 1, 1966.[33] This meant satisfying their elderly constituency, proving to the public at large that federal health insurance could work, and avoiding conflict with the program's powerful opponents in the medical profession—goals that required greater attention to getting hospitals certified than to ensuring their quality.

The rationale behind Medicare was that the elderly could not afford needed care. Chief Medicare officials believed that the way to demonstrate that Medicare could indeed solve that problem was "to pay for care where people get care." Stringent requirements for hospital participation would interfere with the program's goal by disrupting patterns of hospital use and, officials believed, would leave the elderly disappointed and the nation unimpressed.[34] Reinforcing this assessment was some uncertainty, particularly at the highest level of government, about how many people would seek care—and how many beds would be needed—on Medicare's first day.[35] President Lyndon Johnson, who had identified himself with the Medicare program, made it a top proprity that anyone seeking a Medicare-financed hospital stay on July 1 be able to find a bed. Officials purposely chose July 1 as a starting date because its closeness to a holiday made it a low point in hospital occupancy. Similarly, despite administrators' doubts that it would be necessary, the President authorized the use of veterans' and armed services' hospitals for standby beds. In this uncertain and politically charged environment, SSA could not accept a standard of quality that would limit the supply of beds.

Conciliating Medicare's legislative opponents was as important to administrators as satisfying its supporters. Wilbur Cohen, undersecretary of HEW, and his colleagues in SSA believed that unless the people and institutions that had to deliver care would cooperate with government administrators, getting care to the people and ensuring the program's survival would be fraught with difficulty. Administrators felt that an aggressive stance on hospital quality would antagonize hospitals rather than appease them, threatening both the immediate and long-term success of the Medicare program. Despite what a former SSA official described as "good professional backing for closing" many small rural hospitals, he and his colleagues feared that closing them would provoke "a tremendous political problem" from Congress, where rural areas were "over-represented."[36]

In addition to these costs of quality enforcement, Medicare officials throughout the bureaucracy could see several benefits to the alternative. At the top of the administrative hierarchy, officials were committed to Medicare's contribution to a somewhat unrelated policy objective—racial integration.[37] Whether Medicare would require hospitals and other health care institutions to comply with the Civil Rights Act as a condition of payment was a question that Medicare advocates had carefully avoided in legislative debates. Stating that there was never any question that their answer would be yes, strategists explained that they saw to it that their authority was established in the record with a minimum of discussion. When it came time to exercise that authority, top officials wanted to avoid giving hospitals a way out or an excuse to make an uproar. Denying hospitals certification would have let them "off the hook" on civil rights, said one official.[38] As another explained:

If we took them in, they would integrate. If we'd closed them down, they would have said it was because we were forcing them to integrate. Then we'd have a race thing on our hands.[39]

In other words, certifying hospitals would enable HEW to enforce nondiscrimination quietly; denying certification would conflict with that goal.

This did not arouse the attention of officials within SSA's Bureau of Health Insurance (BHI) who were actually writing the Medicare regulations. For them, a primary benefit to avoiding quality enforcement was administrative ease. These officials saw the numerous problems that strict application of standards advocated by PHS would present. What would you do, asked one official, with a hospital that did not meet all the standards—that, for example, met five out of seven requirements and was working hard to meet the other two? "Where is the cut point?"[40] It was their job to find an answer or alternative approach. Because the law provided that health and safety standards could vary by area and class of institution, their first proposal was to develop less stringent standards for hospitals unable to meet JCAH criteria.[41]

To get feedback on this and other policy issues, the Social Security Administration used two advisory structures: ad hoc consultant work groups, put together for particular policy areas and composed of representatives of providers of service, organizations of health professionals, and insurers;[42] and a permanent Health Insurance Benefits Advisory Council (HIBAC), established in the Medicare act to advise administrators on all aspects of policy. Its members were to include people "outstanding in health fields" and "at least one person who is representative of the general public."[43] Although these requirements implied that members would be selected as individuals, policymakers intended to use the Council to involve industry in policymaking, obtaining their acceptance of policy through their participation in its development.[44] Thus most HIBAC members were directly associated with groups of health care institutions or physicians. The constituency to whom public representatives were accountable was less clear. Of four public representatives, one, Nelson Cruikshank, had an identifiable constituency—the AFL–CIO. Cruikshank had worked with Cohen and other Medicare advocates in getting Medicare enacted[45] and seems to have shared administrators' perspective on priorities in its implementation. The following account suggests that in 1965 consumers were as concerned as the bureaucracy with achieving political balance.[46]

The Compromise

From their first consideration of this issue, advisers expressed great concern with the "feasibility" of imposing high standards on all the nation's hospitals. BHI responded with a proposal to use the law's authority to vary health and safety standards by area and class of institution.[47] Their idea was to distinguish hospitals by size, on a rural vs. urban basis, or according to mix of patients (for example, the proportion of patients undergoing surgery), and develop different sets of requirements for each.[48] This would give them a basis for including hospitals that fell below professionally advocated standards. PHS objected to this approach on the grounds that it would freeze unacceptable standards of care in place.[49] BHI officials nevertheless continued to raise this approach for consideration, believing that it was the only way to avoid excluding hospitals.[50] But they too had their difficulties with this approach. They were concerned that in the limited time they had before the program was to start, they would have great difficulty administering a number of sets of standards.[51]

Advisers suggested adopting the JCAH's approach to substandard hospitals: "provisional certification," or certification for a limited time until improvements were made.[52] At first, this approach was explicitly rejected, both because of the PHS emphasis on quality enforcement and BHI doubts about its legality. The latter were explained to HIBAC as follows:

. . . any attempt to model the draft conditions for participation on the Joint Commission's standards has some inherent limitations. For one thing, the Joint Commission's standards are designed to permit the use of subjective "professional judgment" in determining the extent to which a hospital conforms to the general standard. Thus, the Joint Commission recognizes gradations in hospital compliance with its standards and makes allowances for those institutions not fully meeting the standards by providing for "conditional" accreditation. However, it is questionable whether the social security law permits a similar type of flexibility with respect to the conditions for hospital participation. On the contrary, under the hospital insurance program an institution will have to meet all the prescribed requirements applicable to it, and the standards will have to be applied in a way that establishes a legal record upon which the institution could appeal an adverse decision . . . .[53]

As HIBAC debated the issue and developed a consensus behind the commission's "flexible" approach, both PHS and BHI officials resolved their objections. The JCAH approach appealed to advocates of quality improvement because it allowed promotion of a national standard of hospital performance. It was equally acceptable to those concerned with enough beds and industry reaction because it minimized the exclusion of hospitals. As the quality advocates argued to HIBAC:

. . . the Joint Commission continually balances the defects of a hospital against the needs of the community for its services, and . . . the intention is to raise standards rather than to exclude hospitals.[54]

No one mentioned that this reliance on professional discretion would restrict public evaluation of hospital quality and consumer information. An alternative approach—certifying and paying hospitals only for those procedures which they are equipped to perform and publishing their status—was not discussed.

Instead, the result of extensive consultation was a compromise between professional, institutional and administrative points of view. HIBAC recommended and SSA adopted a policy on certification that established a single set of quality criteria for all hospitals, allowed all hospitals to participate without fully conforming to those criteria, and included in the program hospitals falling significantly short of quality standards where their exclusion would restrict beneficiary access to Medicare-financed care.[55] SSA did not explicitly adopt the JCAH's provisional or conditional participation. They achieved the same purpose with fewer punitive implications through the mechanism of "substantial compliance": while all hospitals would officially be required to "meet" in full all of the quality criteria specified in the Medicare law (statutory criteria), a hospital could be found in "substantial compliance" with the conditions that PHS and SSA had developed even with recognized deficiencies

which it is making reasonable plans and efforts to correct and regardless is rendering adequate care without hazard to the health and safety of patients. . . .[56]

In addition, a hospital whose deficiencies were so extensive that it could not be found in substantial compliance could be certified if administrators determined that its exclusion would leave beneficiaries without access to a participating hospital.[57]

Although the conditions of participation included relatively frequent surveys, documentation of deficiencies, and schedules for improvement for deficient hospitals, the guidelines for denial of certification as well as the policy's development emphasized inclusion of hospitals wherever possible. Before recommending that a hospital be denied certification, the guidelines required that the surveyor document consultation with the hospital revealing "no early prospect" for adequate improvement. Second, guidelines specified that termination of a hospital that failed to correct a deficiency would be appropriate when the deficiency jeopardized beneficiary health and safety.[58] Since the hospital was not supposed to be certified at all if health and safety were endangered, this implied that a deficient institution could remain a deficient institution as long as it did not get worse.

This policy was precisely the vehicle BHI needed to achieve its political objectives. It responded to professional pressure to promulgate high standards; to potential beneficiary and hospital pressures to maximize certified beds; and to officials' desires to avoid the administrative difficulties of requiring full compliance. Moreover, it was developed through a process consciously designed to evoke and respond to the concerns of professional and institutional health care interests. Both in substance and in process, SSA's policy on hospital certification reflects a balancing strategy.

Policy Implementation

The implementation of Medicare's conditions of participation also reveals a balancing strategy. Initially, this strategy entailed certifying almost all hospitals, including several that were demonstrably unsafe. Over time, it shaped certification as an "educational" rather than enforcement policy, with considerable sensitivity to the political costs of hospital termination. Furthermore, this sensitivity led SSA to avoid any disruption of the certification process it had developed, either by involving other parties—notably consumers—or by expanding its responsibilities to include overseeing JCAH-accredited institutions. Although there was some political support for both, in the eyes of SSA officials this pressure was never strong enough to risk the peace and political safety of the status quo.

Once advisory groups and the bureaucracy had approved the conditions of participation, administrators began the process of certifying hospitals. Consistent with the objectives behind the conditions, PHS officials reported that

As July 1 approached, there was a notable reluctance to deny certification to any hospital that could meet the statutory requirements.[59]

Another PHS official went further, noting that if even the statutory standards had been rigidly applied, as the law and regulations ostensibly required, some areas would have been left without a participating hospital "for miles."[60] Evaluations of the certification process suggest, however, that even where alternative hospitals were available, inadequate and unsafe hospitals were certified.

Of the roughly 2,700 non-JCAH-accredited hospitals that applied for Medicare certification, less than 8 percent were denied because of noncompliance with the standards.[61] Less than 15 percent were found in substantial compliance with no significant deficiencies; 63 percent of 1,556 hospitals were certified as in substantial compliance with correctable deficiencies; 22 percent or 545 hospitals were found not in substantial compliance but were recommended for special access certification. One-third of the deficient hospitals reportedly fell short of six or more conditions of participation.[62]

How hospitals were classified varied significantly by state, because of variations in the approaches of the state agencies responsible for carrying out the surveys and in the actual quality of hospitals.[63] Approximately three-fourths of the special access hospitals, for example, were in southern states, with the largest concentrations in Texas and Oklahoma.[64]

Although PHS went along with the promulgated approach to certification, their continuing doubts about it appeared in their description of the certification process. Along with references to the "ill defined concept of substantial compliance,"[65] they were particularly dissatisfied with access certification.

It is in this category that we find many of the small, isolated hospitals with minimal nursing services, one or two physicians on the staff, and few, if any, specialized services available. One wonders what health care function these facilities really serve . . . . In one instance, we discovered a real function for such a hospital—during a heavy rainstorm all the power and water in the community were cut off, and the hospital, with its emergency power and water supply, served as the community center.[66]

Evaluations of the certification process, conducted by both the Medicare program and the General Accounting Office, provide evidence for doubt. The first were undertaken by PHS and BHI officials in 1967 and 1968.[67] Review teams reported the certification "in substantial compliance" of hospitals violating the regulations' explicit requirement that there be no hazards to health and safety. Two states explained the inclusion of hospitals with fire hazards as a response to the "initial pressures" to get beds into the program.[68] In Arizona, identified as a state with "weak certification operations," a hospital certified in substantial compliance was described by the State Health Department's Planning and Construction Division as "so rickety and unstable that the floors bend and squeak when walked upon."[69] The state files revealed other hospitals with severe fire hazards, including one hospital in which "it would be virtually impossible to evacuate to safety the patients on the second floor."[70]

In 1968 the General Accounting Office (GAO) investigated certification in Texas, where problems of compliance with Medicare standards appeared most serious.[71] In the program's first year, the Texas state agency reportedly recommended termination of forty-two hospitals. In thirty of these, there were deficiencies related to statutory requirements, including one for twenty-four-hour supervision of care by a registered nurse.[72] Other hospitals were found "deficient in such areas as fire protection, sanitation in the dietary department and operating room, safe-guarding of drugs, and the investigation, control, and prevention of infection."[73]

Most of the 42 hospitals were located in rural communities having populations of less than 7,000. For the fiscal year ended June 30, 1967, over 7,400 Medicare patients had been admitted to these hospitals and the related payments for services rendered totaled over $1.5 million. GAO believes that most of these patients could have been accommodated in other hospitals that met the standards for participation in the program.[74]

The certification of hospitals that did not meet Medicare's standards is no surprise, given SSA's concerns at the program's start. But what happened to them later reveals the continuation of SSA's balancing strategy. Although some of the hospitals described above ultimately had their certification withdrawn or terminated,[75] SSA was very reluctant to use this authority. Officials continued to view hospital certification as a highly political issue, in which the costs of quality enforcement significantly outweighed the benefits. The GAO report mentioned above was addressed to BHI's delays in acting on state agency recommendations that hospitals be terminated. Between August 1966 and August 1967 the Texas agency recommended termination of forty-two hospitals. The BHI regional office submitted thirty-nine of the forty-two to the regional office of PHS' Division of Medical Care Administration, which concurred in the state agency's recommendation. The GAO reported that by April 1968, SSA had resolved the status of only sixteen of these hospitals.[76]

GAO attributed this delay to the extensive documentation SSA required of the state agency's case against the hospital, without any time limits for the correction of deficiencies identified.[77] Initially, BHI required that the state agency describe the consultations it had offered the hospitals, notify the hospitals of the termination recommendations, and document the availability of other certified hospitals in the same area. But following SSA's resolution of its first termination case, the agency issued new instructions for termination proceedings. According to the GAO,

the effect of the September 1967 instructions was to further increase the proof required to be developed by a state agency with regard to (1) the continuing existence of a hospital's deficiencies and (2) the extent of the state agency's consultative efforts to correct the deficiencies. These instructions, however, included no requirement for establishing specific time limits within which hospitals would be required to meet the statutory and regulatory conditions of participation.[78]

In interviews, BHI officials acknowledged their emphasis on extensive documentation and related it to their concern that any termination action be unassailable in court. No termination was undertaken, officials explained, unless the agency was certain it would win on appeal.[79] This concern with winning is not unique to SSA and is another indication of the agency's concern with support from the outside world.[80] The kind of documentation winning required, however, is evidence of its specific strategy to ensure support—an "educational" rather than enforcement approach. The Florida state agency, complaining about BHI's termination policy, proposed to its program review team that certification standards be written as minimal requirements so that "termination proposals would involve clearcut cases that hearing examiners could not rule on adversely to SSA." They believed

that where physical plant deficiencies exist to the extent that health and safety are placed in jeopardy, the facility should be terminated for that fact alone, and it should not be necessary to document all the other deficiencies.[81]

The survey team explained to the agency why this idea was unacceptable.

The conditions are intended, in part, as guides for upgrading medical services and . . . to frame them in terms of solid cases for termination would result in weakening our efforts to encourage higher standards; in light of this, the need to make a good case for termination involves pointing out to the hearing examiner why a particular requirement is essential.[82]

The obstacles this posed to termination of even inadequate hospitals is demonstrated by the Florida case. By 1968, the Florida state agency had recommended that ten extended care facilities and four hospitals be terminated. In response to the initial pressure to maximize Medicare beds, Florida certified a number of old and hazardous facilities but intended to phase them out of the program "at the earliest opportunity." SSA's consultation requirements stood in the way of this plan. The program review team reported that the state agency was

not suggesting expensive improvements in physical plant which would bring the old buildings into full compliance with the conditions of participation and prolong their existence. This approach to marginal providers results in an apparent lack of effort on the part of the State agency to assist the facilities to upgrade, and absence of documentation on such consultation to complete a case for termination according to instructions.[83]

Thus the educational approach meant the receipt of Medicare funds and provision of questionable benefits by inadequate or unsafe hospitals.

Responding to this criticism from the GAO, SSA explained that its policy assured "an active influence leading to improvement in the quality of hospital care." Claiming that most situations where termination was considered did not immediately endanger patient health and safety, they argued that consultation led to upgrading and avoided a disruptive, administratively costly "in-out-in effect."[84] But the evidence challenges these explanations, indicating that consultation rather than enforcement meant continuing deficiencies. Hospitals certified in substantial compliance had no incentive to achieve full compliance. Pointing this out, the Oregon state agency asked for BHI guidance

in situations where they will be continually citing the same deficiencies and where either the institution has made no effort to correct the deficiency or it is just impossible to correct the deficiency.[85]

Termination did not seem a "suitable alternative in all of these cases."[86]

The GAO's solution to this problem was to recommend incorporating time limits for the correction of deficiencies,[87] but a former SSA official observed that the difficulty was more fundamental. Even with time limits, he said, the agency would have to decide what to do when the time was up.[88] The attitudes and sensitivities that made certification what one official described as "an improvement not a policing policy"[89] would persist.

Like the development of substantial compliance, the educational approach was sensitive to beneficiary and hospital attitudes toward quality enforcement. In explaining why noncomplying hospitals were certified in Texas and elsewhere when alternatives were available within fifteen to thirty-five miles, SSA argued that "many beneficiaries are reluctant to be hospitalized outside their community," even if only in the next town. Furthermore, termination would disrupt physician-patient relationships unless alternative hospital affiliations could be arranged. Describing the limited mobility and adaptability of the elderly, SSA explained:

Our approach in Texas was therefore influenced by the realization that application of the Medicare health and safety requirements to all of the nation's hospitals, the very largest as well as the smallest, must, of necessity, be tempered by the recognition and understanding of the diverse patterns for the provision of health care services that exist in different sections of the country. While the upgrading of health care is a major program objective, SSA must recognize the need, particularly in the early stages of Medicare, to build public confidence in the program. We are concerned that the almost simultaneous termination of relatively large numbers of hospitals, that over the years have become the principal places to which the community turns when severe illness strikes, could produce adverse community reaction ultimately resulting in a weakening of hospital health and safety requirements and thereby leading to a lowering of the quality of health care provided to significant segments of the population.[90]

A BHI official responsible for certification explained how beneficiary and institutional concerns merged to create political problems for the agency.[91] Think about a small town hospital, he said, owned by the town's two beloved physicians and staffed with licensed practical nurses, "nice old ladies whom everybody loves." Without supervision by a registered nurse, the hospital would be out of compliance with Medicare's statutory requirements. The community, said this official, knows little of nursing requirements and is unaware that "nice little old ladies" do not know what to do if someone hemorrhages. All the community sees is that in their own hospital people know and care about them; at the hospital thirty miles away they would be strangers.

If you terminate this hospital, the BHI official explained, the community is up in arms. The local paper is filled without outrage, demanding some action from their representative in Congress. Asked to demonstrate his influence in Washington, the congressman is hard put to refuse. The agency's explanation may carry no weight; after all, if the congressman needs hospitalization, "he can go to Bethesda."[92]

Because of sensitivity to this possibility, SSA kept tight central control over the termination process. In contrast to certification decisions, until 1974 final decisions on termination were made in the central rather than the regional offices.[93] PHS officials participated in regional recommendations, but had a limited role at the top. According to a participating PHS official, SSA did not trust PHS to be politically sensitive. "They were afraid that if they gave us a veto, we would stand firm." PHS officials, sometimes asked by BHI for support on a termination action, reported offering to push the issues to the top of their hierarchy if BHI had trouble with its superiors in SSA. But BHI never wanted that much "help." This official recalled termination actions going all the way to the Social Security commissioner, who would reply: "Don't terminate unless you get the approval of the congressman." "I learned from SSA," said this official, "that you can't go into Arkansas, the state of Wilbur Mills, and throw out a hospital."[94]

The thrust of this perspective, however, was not failure to act. Just as they compromised with health professionals on the promulgation of standards, SSA officials responded to professional evaluations of inadequacies, and following the procedures outlined above, did terminate some hospitals.[95] As one official described it, they "turned the screw and watched for a reaction."[96] They began with hospitals that failed to meet the statutory twenty-four hour registered nurse (RN) requirement and other standards, including "physical environment." Forty-two of the 116 hospitals terminated as of 1974 were in Texas, the state with the greatest number of substandard facilities.[97] Despite SSA's caution, they got a reaction from Texas Congressman Omar Burleson, in whose district many of the hospitals were located. In 1970 he introduced and Congress passed an amendment to the law providing that the secretary could waive (for five years) the requirement for twenty-four hour RN coverage, for any one-year period for small rural hospitals certified in the access category.[98] BHI and PHS contracted for a study to find a more permanent solution to nursing shortages,[99] the objective of which, said one official, would be the "highest standards consistent with reality." In the meantime, the Burleson amendment was regarded as an "impediment to termination."[100]

Maintaining the Compromise

To SSA officials, this congressional response represented the political limits on quality enforcement. But their reactions to proposals that could alter the limits reveal SSA's commitment to preserving the political balance it had already achieved. Reactions ranging from reluctance to resistance were reflected in SSA's responses to consumer advocates seeking disclosure of hospital surveys, and to HIBAC and consumer advocate proposals to have government take full responsibility for hospital quality.

Although they argued that communities objected to quality enforcement, SSA officials resisted attempts to expand information that could change that situation. In 1970 Mal Schechter, consumer-oriented editor of *Hospital Practice*, sought to obtain the Medicare survey report on Boston City Hospital. The hospital had been disaccredited by JCAH, which clearly suggested inadequacies, and yet had been certified as in substantial compliance with Medicare requirements. SSA refused to make the survey available.[101] At the same time the agency was opposing an amendment proposed by the Senate Finance Committee to require public disclosure of Medicare surveys.[102]

SSA perceived these proposals as likely to disrupt their certification arrangements. They believed that their approach to certification adequately protected consumers and avoided antagonizing hospitals. Publicity would disrupt this arrangement, they believed, without increasing quality. Asked to comment on public disclosure, officials explained their concerns. A senior official argued that survey data were not designed for public understanding and sometimes included extensive material on minor deficiencies. "What's the point," he asked, "of upsetting a community with unimportant deficiencies?"[103] Schechter quoted Commissioner Ball's observation on the consequences of such disruption: "Adverse public reaction could severely hamper an institution's effort to maintain patient loads while effectuating needed improvements."[104] An official more directly involved in the certification process expressed another potential cost of publicity. Knowledge that surveys would be published, he claimed, could discourage the surveyor from making negative evaluations and thereby destroy the integrity of the certification process.[105]

SSA believed that they had achieved an effective compromise of interests and wanted to maintain it. This engendered a narrow perspective, as demonstrated by their behavior after Congress enacted the disclosure provision. Some involved officials reported that the new provision was inadequately publicized.[106] But even one who argued that the agency welcomed and tried to promote consumer activity gave evidence of the contrary. Commenting that the agency's fear that publicity would inhibit surveyors had proved groundless, he claimed that SSA would be delighted to see an upsurge in expression of consumer opinions and had, in fact, informed "everybody"—state agencies, fiscal agents, district offices— about the new requirement. But when asked whether SSA had informed beneficiaries, he replied that they had not. First suggesting that the agency could be faulted for this "flaw" in its approach, he went on to justify it with arguments like those used to oppose the provision in the first place: encouraging consumer complaints would produce a rash of complaints about "cold hamburgers."[107] The possibility that informing beneficiaries of a hospital's capabilities and deficiencies might keep them from using unsafe hospitals was apparently not entertained. Maintaining a compromise based on the fact that consumers were ignorant meant keeping them that way.

Another example of SSA's desire not to disrupt its political compromise was its reluctance to expand its authority to oversee hospital quality. Although its standards applied only to non-JCAH-accredited hospitals, Medicare's evaluation of hospital quality also brought to light problems in JCAH-accredited hospitals. State agencies, HIBAC, and consumer advocates therefore pressed SSA to withdraw the Medicare law's delegation of authority to the Joint Commission.

State agencies reported that Medicare standards were more stringently applied than JCAH's.[108] As a result, hospitals attempted to evade Medicare controls by becoming accredited. This produced inconsistencies, compounded by variations in the law. Accreditation did not ensure certification of extended care facilities (ECFs); thus a state agency could deny certification as an ECF to part of a JCAH-accredited facility it found unsafe. The beds could then become part of an accredited, and therefore certified, hospital. A HIBAC subcommittee reported a similar situation with clinical laboratories.[109] A laboratory could be denied licensure under the 1967 Clinical Laboratories Improvement Act but certified for Medicare participation as part of a JCAH-accredited hospital.

Distressed by this situation, state agencies recommended legislation that would allow them to survey participating JCAH hospitals that had received one year provisional accreditation.[110] In 1969, responding to the information state agencies had provided, HIBAC went further.

Initially, Medicare's reliance on JCAH accreditation standards and certification procedures helped the new federal program win the acceptance and support of the health professions and was beneficial to both the government and the health professions. The Council believes, however, that it is inappropriate to continue statutory delegation to a private agency of all the government's authority to safeguard quality of care paid for by a government program. The authority to establish policy on minimum quality should be retained by the government.

Quality standards under Medicare should not be controlled by a private agency's standards. Furthermore, the power of oversight and assurance that standards are applied adequately in individual situations should and must remain within both the responsibility and authority of the government.[111]

Accordingly, HIBAC recommended legislation to remove the JCAH ceiling on standards, relying on accreditation as evidence of compliance only where JCAH standards were equal to or higher than the secretary's, and authorizing state agency surveys and certification recommendations on JCAH-accredited hospitals.[112]

Both PHS and BHI officials working with state agencies recall having drafted and "sent up" amendments on this order,[113] but they were never pressed by senior BHI or SSA officials or adopted by HEW. BHI Director Thomas Tierney told HIBAC that the agency was designing a study to compare Medicare certification with subsequent JCAH accreditation, but even this was apparently not undertaken.[114] Although discussions with JCAH reportedly upgraded their performance,[115] no change in the SSA–JCAH relationship was sought. Asked to explain this, officials at lower levels in BHI attributed three concerns to their superiors: (1) action would constitute an attack on organized medicine; (2) the monetary cost of surveying all hospitals would be enormous; and (3) political heat would increase with full responsibility. To paraphrase their views on the last of these: "The pressure related to quality regulation was bad enough; for large, well-known hospitals, it would be even worse."[116]

Further evidence of this attitude comes from the results of a 1971 legal challenge to Medicare's delegation of authority to the JCAH.[117] Having failed to prevent the accreditation of two municipal hospitals that they found dangerous, organizations of elderly citizens asked HEW to review the hospitals for compliance with Medicare standards. BHI denied the request on the grounds that JCAH-accredited hospitals were not subject to HEW review. When the hospitals' inadequacies persisted and the elderly could get redress from neither JCAH nor HEW under existing law, they sued the department on the grounds that its delegation of authority to the Joint Commission was unconstitutional.

A lawyer for the plaintiff reported that the department did not make an active defense in the suit, leaving it to JCAH, who asked to be a defendant. Although this lawyer was not convinced that the elderly groups would win the case, BHI officials apparently felt that the odds were on the side of the plaintiffs. JCAH, for whom the law suit was very expensive, shared that point of view. Thus "everybody was looking for a way out"—a change in the law that would alter the delegation of authority and moot the court case.[118] Accordingly, the Senate Finance Committee staff, working with the agency and JCAH, drafted an appropriate amendment. As enacted, the amendment removed the JCAH ceiling on standards, authorized state agencies to inspect and evaluate accredited hospitals on a sample basis and in response to complaints, and required institutions to authorize the commission to release its accreditation survey reports to the secretary on request.[119] According to one official, this "halfway position" responded to the problem while avoiding the major administrative and political implications of a vast expansion of SSA's survey responsibilities.[120] The Finance Committee report emphasized the continuing role of the commission, and characterized the amendments as intended to "validate" the JCAH process.[121]

Officials described their implementation of the provision in terms of similar sensitivities.[122] One official explained that the agency had no basis and no desire to encourage "squealing" on JCAH hospitals, nor to induce a rash of "cold hamburger" complaints. Although they reported a change in one hospital's certification status on the basis of complaints, BHI officials did not expect much activity in this area.

They reported more activity on the sample surveys, the first of which revealed thirty-six of sixty-five hospitals, some of them large and reputable institutions, out of compliance with the National Fire Protection Association's Life Safety Code. BHI notified the hospitals that their accredited status no longer made them automatically in compliance and informed Congress and JCAH of the "problem area." But officials reported that BHI continued to avoid taking over full certification responsibility.[123]

Conclusion

When SSA had to make a decision on hospital quality enforcement in 1965, they assessed the reactions of interested parties to alternative actions, weighed their political consequences, and developed an acceptable compromise. Over the next ten years they evaluated hospital quality in a way that would maintain that compromise. This strategy is apparent in both the policy process and its outcomes. To ensure that any action they took would find support or at least acceptance, SSA consulted with affected parties, long maintained central control over termination decisions, and continually evaluated political interest in their actions. Out of these activities, they developed an "educational" approach to certification, terminating hospitals cautiously and infrequently, and emphasizing improvement of deficiencies rather than imposing sanctions. They perceived as disruptive proposals to involve consumers in certification evaluations or to expand their certification task. SSA has viewed their compromise as successful and has seen so reason to change.

SSA's strategy of balancing pressures originated in Medicare's legislative history. In their thirty-year effort to get some form of federal health insurance enacted, Wilbur Cohen and his colleagues developed a view of the world as comprised of Medicare supporters and opponents. Their approach to administration was to satisfy the former without antagonizing the latter, and to do so in a way that was easy to administer. In 1965 this meant tempering their desire to ignore quality with recognition of professional concern that Medicare upgrade hospital quality. The administrative mechanisms they developed to implement this compromise gave them room for the continual consultation and political evaluation they believed necessary to maintain it.

SSA perceived this strategy as the best way to serve their elderly constituency. They believed that a different approach, like the one PHS advocated, for example, would lead to Medicare's political demise. Although they continued to believe this, the rationale behind it became less important over time. In its place came a vested interest in the status quo. Administrators tried to avoid controversy. Believing that the way they did things was the "best" way to do things, they devoted attention and energy to maintaining the 1965 arrangements. Proposals to change or expand were perceived as disruptions, not opportunities, that would create unwanted political and administrative problems.

The officials who devised this strategy believe it has been a political success, and has upgraded the quality of hospital care at the same time. I do not intend to challenge these viewpoints. I have not reviewed the evidence on overall hospital performance and find it difficult if not impossible to outline what might have happened politically if administrators had done something different. But whether successful or not, the balancing strategy has had both quality and political costs that cannot be ignored. Because the "educational" approach allows inadequate and even unsafe hospitals to participate in Medicare, beneficiaries cannot depend upon hospital certification to assure them of proper care. Furthermore, this approach means expending public funds to perpetuate hospitals that, based on the quality of care they provide, should perhaps go out of business. These facts must be considered alongside improved performance of many hospitals in evaluating Medicare certification.

Equally important have been the political consequences of the "educational" approach. By keeping measurement of hospital quality a matter of administrative discretion, Medicare has suppressed consumer and local political evaluation of hospitals. The elderly who sued HEW believed that removal of a hospital's accreditation or certification would force communities to recognize and do something about unsafe hospitals. SSA has prevented this both by certifying inadequate hospitals and by resisting the publication of the quality surveys. By keeping the public uninformed, the balancing strategy has thus reinforced the configuration of political interests on which it was originally based.

Notes

1. For the evolution of government regulation of hospital quality, see Anne R. Somers, *Hospital Regulation: The Dilemma of Public Policy* (Princeton, N.J.: Industrial Relations Section, Princeton University, 1969), chapter 6; John W. Cashman, Pearl Bierman and Beverlee A. Myers, "The Why of the Medicare Conditions of Participation," adapted from talk given by Ms. Bierman

at the Federal Bar Association Briefing Conference on Medicare, Washington, D.C., April 20, 1967 (typewritten).

2. 42 U.S.C. sec. 1395x(e).

3. For congressional intent, see excerpts from *Report of the Committee on Finance, United States Senate, to accompany H.R. 6675*, pp. 28–29; excerpts from *Report of the Committee on Ways and Means on H.R. 6675*, pp. 25–26, both in New Members Background Book, Part I, for Health Insurance Benefits Advisory Council (HIBAC), 1968. For a description of HIBAC and its role in Medicare implementation, see the section of this chapter entitled "Policy Objectives."

4. The Joint Commission is sponsored by the American Medical Association, the American Hospital Association, the American College of Physicians, and the American College of Surgeons. For its history see Feather Davis Hair, "Hospital Accreditation: A Developmental Study of the Social Control of Institutions" (Ph.D. dissertation, Vanderbilt University, 1972).

5. 42 U.S.C. sec. 1395bb and sec. 1395x(e) (8). The law included some exceptions to these provisions. Even accredited hospitals had to be reviewed for compliance with statutory utilization review requirements. These provisions are found in 42 U.S.C. sec. 1395z and sec. 1395bb. Interviews with former HEW officials indicate the appeal of these provisions to Medicare strategists. They were amenable to administrative arrangements that prevented the secretary from appearing the "czar of medicine" while still allowing some quality regulation. Accordingly, the administration's legislative proposals throughout the early sixties included a JCAH role. Due to some initial concern about the constitutionality of delegating authority, however, 1961 legislative language required that the secretary find that accreditation provided reasonable assurance that Medicare quality criteria were met before deeming accredited institutions in compliance. This requirement was absent from subsequent legislative proposals. Wilbur Cohen's chief adviser on this and other legal questions was Alanson Willcox, who worked for the AHA prior to his appointment in 1961 as HEW general counsel. For the AMA pressure on this issue, see "Suit Challenges Delegation of Medicare Standards to JCAH," *Hospital Practice* 7 (February 1972): 199. For legislative history, see U.S., Department of Health, Education, and Welfare, Social Security Administration, *Background on Medicare 1957–1962; Reports, Studies and Congressional Considerations on Health Legislation*, 2 vols. 85th–87th Congress.

6. See Hair, "Hospital Accreditation."

7. Ibid., p. 40, reprinted with permission.

8. Cashman, Bierman, and Myers, "Medicare Conditions of Participation," pp. 1–2, reprinted with permission.

9. For a discussion of consumers' inability to judge the quality of medical care, see Avedis Donabedian, *A Guide to Medical Care Administration*, vol. 2 (New York: American Public Health Association, 1969), pp. 109–10.

10. See Hair, "Hospital Accreditation," expecially pp. 188–90; Madison D. Brown, M.D. (Associate Director, AHA), "Accreditation of Hospitals," *Hospital Progress* 46 (January 1965): 95–97; John W. Cashman and Beverlee A. Myers, "Medicare: Standards of Service in a New Program—Licensure, Certification, Accreditation," *American Journal of Public Health* 57 (July 1967): 1108: "The key element here is that standards define a certain capacity for quality and not the quality itself. We assume that, given this capacity a level of quality will result. And experience informs us that without this capacity, achievement of quality is difficult, if not impossible."

11. See Avedis Donabedian, *Medical Care Administration*, pp. 2–4.

12. See Patrick O'Donoghue, *Evidence about the Effects of Health Care Regulation* (Denver, Colo.: Spectrum Research, Inc., 1974), pp. 85–86; Hair, "Hospital Accreditation" especially pp. 188–90 and p. 357 with citations; and "The Role of Standards," in Arthur D. Little, Inc., "Study of Special Certification Standards for Limited Service Rural Hospitals," Final Report, Contract HSM 110–72–375, C–74840, June 1974, pp. 5–7.

13. William Worthington and Laurens H. Silver, "Regulation of Quality of Care in Hospitals: The Need for Change," from a symposium, "Health Care: Part I" appearing in *Law and Contemporary Problems* 35:2 (Spring 1970), 305–33, published by the Duke University School of Law, Durham, N.C., copyright 1970, 1971, by Duke University; and "Suit Challenges Delegation of Medicare Standards to JCAH," pp. 186–208.

14. "Memorandum of Points and Authorities in Support of Plaintiffs' Motion for Summary Judgment," Self-Help for the Elderly, et al. v. Elliot Richardson, et al., Civil Action No. 2016-71, in the U.S. District Court for the District of Columbia, p. 15 (typewritten).

15. Worthington and Silver, "Quality of Care," n. 2 p. 306, reprinted with permission.

16. Timothy S. Robinson, "Hospital Details Cost of Edict," *Washington Post*, December 4, 1975, p. B1.

17. See Worthington and Silver, "Quality of Care."

18. Ibid., n. 1, p. 305, reprinted with permission.

19. M.N. Zald and F.D. Hair, "The Social Control of General Hospitals," in Basil S. Georgopoulos, ed., *Organization Research on Health Institutions* (Ann Arbor, Mich.: Institute for Social Research, University of Michigan, 1972), pp. 68–71.

20. Ibid. For a description of problems in proprietary hospitals, see Edwin P. Hoyt, *Condition Critical: Our Hospital Crisis* (New York: Holt, Rinehart, and Winston, 1966), chapter 4.

21. Anne R. Somers, *Hospital Regulation*, p. 106. AHA data on accredited hospitals in 1965 include a small number of hospitals with fewer than twenty-five beds, suggesting that such accreditation did sometimes occur. *Hospitals, Journal of the American Hospital Association* 40 (August 1, 1966):472.

22. AHA data on accredited hospitals in 1967, 1968, and 1969 reveal far fewer accredited hospitals with fewer than twenty-five beds than in the 25–49

bed category. *Hospitals, Journal of the American Hospital Association* 42 (August 1, 1968): 468; 43 (August 1, 1969): 495; 44 (August 1, 1970): 496. These findings are suggestive more than proof of hospitals' ability to meet standards, for other factors affect both accreditation and the statistics.

23. Background Book for HIBAC, 1965, p. IVA2; and Cashman and Myers, "Medicare," p. 1114.

24. See pp. 16-17.

25. Hair, "Hospital Accreditation," p. 406, supported by Arthur D. Little, Inc., "Special Certification Standards," pp. 1-4, reprinted with permission.

26. For a discussion of the evolution of hospital quality and quality control, see Herman M. Somers and Anne R. Somers, *Medicare and the Hospitals; Issues and Prospects*, Studies in Social Economics (Washington, D.C.: The Brookings Institution, 1967), pp. 76-80.

27. The law did require that all hospitals meet state licensure requirements where they existed, but, with few exceptions, these requirements were significantly inferior to JCAH standards. See Anne R. Somers, pp. 108-15, who speaks of a "near-vacuum" of hospital regulation at the state level.

28. This compromise is discussed in Herman M. Somers and Anne R. Somers, *Medicare and the Hospitals*, pp. 85-88 and 91-93.

29. See "Health Insurance for Aged Persons," in Social Security Administration, *Background on Medicare*, p. 73.

30. Interviews with former HEW and PHS officials and "Background of Draft Standards for Hospitals," staff memorandum for HIBAC, HIBAC Agenda Book, November 12-13, 1965. The work groups also included representatives of the Welfare Administration, responsible for implementing Medicaid.

31. Dr. John Cashman of PHS, presenting draft standards to HIBAC, HIBAC minutes, Meeting I:Session 2, November 13, 1965, pp. 14-15. By decision of the Council (I:1, November 12, 1965, p. 6), HIBAC minutes are summaries rather than verbatim records. Quotes are therefore from summaries, not direct.

32. Interviews with former PHS and SSA officials; HIBAC materials, Consultant Work Groups, summary of meeting, September 13-14, 1965, p. 2; "Background of Draft Standards for Hospitals," in HIBAC Agenda Book, November 12-13, 1965, pp. 1-2; HIBAC minutes, I:2, November 13, 1965, pp. 14-15.

33. Interviews with former HEW and SSA officials.

34. Ibid.

35. The following account comes from interviews with former HEW and SSA officials.

36. Interviews with former HEW and SSA officials.

37. This account comes from interviews with former HEW and SSA officials.

38. Interview with former SSA official.

39. Interview with former HEW official. A former civil rights official recalled that Medicare administrators only became committed to immediate

desegregation after a press campaign launched by civil rights activists; here as elsewhere, they were responding to political pressure.

40. Interview with present and former BHI officials.

41. Interview with present and former BHI officials, and BHI presentation to Consultant Work Groups, summary of September 13–14, 1965, meeting, p. 5.

42. The Consultant Work Group on Provider Participation, for example, included representatives of the AHA, AMA, National Medical Association, American Nurses Association, American Osteopathic Association, American Osteopathic Hospital Association, American Psychological Association, American State and Territorial Health Officials, Blue Cross Association, insurance industry, and JCAH.

43. 42 U.S.C. sec. 1395dd.

44. Interviews with former HEW and BHI officials.

45. For Cruikshank's important role in Medicare's legislative history, see Richard Harris, *A Sacred Trust* (Baltimore, Md.: Penguin Books, Pelican Books, 1969), pp. 71–73.

46. For insights on consumer perspectives in Medicare's early days, I am indebted to Mal Schechter, personal communication, and Mal Schechter, "Medicare's Secret Data," in U.S., Congress, House, Committee on Ways and Means, *National Health Insurance Proposals, Hearings*, 92nd Cong., 1st sess., 1971, pp. 3026–28.

47. Consultant Work Groups, summary of meeting, September 13–14, 1965.

48. Interview with BHI official.

49. Interview with former PHS official.

50. HIBAC, "Background of Draft Standards for Hospitals," and HIBAC minutes, I:2, November 13, 1965, p. 15.

51. Interview with BHI official.

52. Consultant Work Groups, summary of meeting, September 13–14, 1965.

53. HIBAC, "Background of Draft Standards for Hospitals," pp. 1–2.

54. HIBAC minutes, I:2, November 13, 1965, pp. 15–16.

55. Ibid., p. 16, and HIBAC minutes, III:3, December 19, 1965, pp. 36–38.

56. For requirements see HIBAC minutes, III:3, December 19, 1965, pp. 36–38; "Conditions of Participation for Hospitals," draft, December 16, 1965, HIBAC Agenda Book, December 17–19, 1965, pp. iv–viii and 20 C.F.R. 405.1003–405.1011.

57. "Conditions for Participation," p. viii and 20 C.F.R. sec. 405.1010.

58. "Conditions for Participation," pp. vii–viii and 20 C.F.R. sec. 405.1007 and sec. 405.1009.

59. Cashman and Myers, "Medicare," p. 1109, reprinted with permission.

60. Interview with former PHS official.

61. This percentage did not include a number of nonaccredited hospitals that either did not apply or withdrew their applications when it appeared they could not meet the standards and be certified. Cashman and Myers, "Medicare," p. 1114.

62. Ibid., pp. 1114–15.

63. Ibid., p. 1114.

64. "Recertification of Access Hospitals," Staff Memorandum for HIBAC, HIBAC Agenda Book, September 16–17, 1967.

65. Cashman and Myers, "Medicare," p. 1114, reprinted with permission.

66. Ibid., p. 1113, reprinted with permission.

67. This information comes from "Summary of Program Review Findings and State Agency Recommendations," Staff Report for Subcommittee on Hospital and Extended Care Services, Committee on the Evaluation of Delivery and Utilization of Services (CEDUS), HIBAC; and Selected State Reports; both in HIBAC, Task Force on Hospital and Extended Care Services, notebook, September 9–12, 1968.

68. Selected State Reports: Ohio Report, p. 5; Florida Report, p. 4.

69. Ibid., Arizona Report, p. 3.

70. Ibid., pp. 3–4. This particular hospital was terminated on March 9, 1970.

71. See U.S., General Accounting Office, *Need for Timely Action in Resolving Problems Affecting the Eligibility of Hospitals under the Medicare Program*, B–164031(4), Social Security Administration, Department of Health, Education, and Welfare, Report to the Congress by the Comptroller General of the United States, Washington, D.C., December 27, 1968.

72. Another violation was utilization review. See Chapter 3.

73. General Accounting Office, *Need for Timely Action*, p. 9.

74. Ibid., p. 1.

75. See "Involuntarily Terminated Facilities (by Region) as of May 1, 1974," available from BHI's Division of State Operations.

76. General Accounting Office, *Need for Timely Action*, p. 1.

77. Ibid., pp. 23–25; pp. 27–31.

78. Ibid., pp. 23–25.

79. Interviews with BHI officials.

80. For this general phenomenon, see Roger G. Noll, *Reforming Regulation: An Evaluation of the Ash Council Proposals*, Studies in the Regulation of Economic Activity (Washington, D.C.: The Brookings Institution, 1971), pp. 40–42.

81. Selected State Reports: Florida Report, p. 3.

82. Ibid., p. 3.

83. Ibid., pp. 3–4.

84. General Accounting Office, *Need for Timely Action*, pp. 39–40.

85. Selected State Reports: Oregon Report, p. 3; see also General Accounting Office, *Need for Timely Action*, pp. 28–29.

86. Selected State Reports: Oregon Report, p. 3.

87. General Accounting Office, *Need for Timely Action*, pp. 32–33.

88. Interview.

89. Interview with official in BHI's Division of State Operations.

90. SSA response in General Accounting Office, *Need for Timely Action*, appendix 2, pp. 2–5. Similar statement in staff report to HIBAC, HIBAC Agenda Book, April 27–28, 1968.

91. Interview with BHI official in Division of State Operations.

92. For a similar view, see Somers and Somers, *Medicare and the Hospitals*, pp. 91-92.

93. Interview with BHI officials in Division of State Operations.

94. Interview with former PHS official.

95. As of May 1974, SSA had terminated 116 hospitals (total includes 26 hospitals readmitted or closed). "Involuntarily Terminated Facilities (by Region) as of May 1, 1974," available from BHI's Division of State Operations.

96. Interview with former SSA official.

97. "Involuntarily Terminated Facilities."

98. Explained to HIBAC, HIBAC minutes, clearance draft, XL:1, June 18, 1971, p. 12 in HIBAC Agenda Book, July 23-24, 1971, and "Conditions for Participation," p. 13, HIBAC Agenda Book, June 18-19, 1971.

99. HIBAC minutes, clearance draft, XL:1, June 18, 1971, pp. 12-13, and interview with PHS official.

100. Interview with BHI official. "Substantial compliance" has persisted despite changes in the Medicare regulations in 1974. The changes, BHI officials explained, were a response to Senate Finance Committee criticism but served public relations purposes and reportedly had no operational consequences.

101. "'Top Secret' at SSA: Why?" *Hospital Practice* (February 1972): 195-96. See also Mal Schechter, "Medicare's Secret Data," pp. 3026-28.

102. "'Top Secret' at SSA: Why?" pp. 195-96.

103. Interview with SSA official.

104. "'Top Secret' at SSA: Why?" p. 196.

105. Interview with official in BHI's Division of State Operations.

106. Interview with officials in BHI's Division of State Operations.

107. Interview with official in BHI's Division of State Operations.

108. "Summary of Program Review Findings," CEDUS, HIBAC, p. 5, and Selected State Reports: Arkansas Report, p. 6; Florida Report, p. 10.

109. Task Force on Laboratory Services—Preliminary Report, CEDUS, HIBAC, CEDUS Agenda Book, November 2, 1968, pp. 12-13.

110. Summary of Program Review Findings, CEDUS, HIBAC, p. 5.

111. U.S., Department of Health, Education, and Welfare, Social Security Administration, Bureau of Health Insurance, *Health Insurance Benefits Advisory Council Annual Report on Medicare: Covering the Period July 1, 1966 to December 31, 1967* (Washington, D.C.: July 1969), pp. 10-11.

112. Ibid., pp. 11-12.

113. Interviews with BHI and PHS officials.

114. HIBAC minutes, XVIII:1, March 2, 1968, p. 6. Officials interviewed did not recall this study being done. A senior official in the Division of State Operations interviewed in 1973 said he did not know whether Medicare or JCAH was more stringent in its application of standards.

115. HIBAC minutes, XXI, September 21, 1968, p. 12, and interviews with PHS official.

116. Interviews with officials in BHI's Division of State Operations.

117. Information on the suit comes from "Memorandum of Points and Authorities in Support of Plaintiffs' Motion for Summary Judgment," Self-Help for the Elderly, et al. v. Elliot Richardson, et al., Civil Action No. 2016–71, in the U.S. District Court for the District of Columbia. Also "Suit Challenges Delegation of Medicare Standards to JCAH," pp. 186ff., and interview with a lawyer for the plaintiffs.

118. Interview with present and former BHI officials.

119. P.L. 92–603, Section 244, enacted October 30, 1972. See also U.S., Congress, Senate, Committee on Finance, Excerpt from Senate Report 92–1230, *Report of the Committee on Finance to Accompany H.R.1, the Social Security Amendments of 1972*, IV, Provisions Relating to Medicare–Medicaid and Maternal and Child Health, 92d Cong., 2d sess., 1972, pp. 289–91.

120. Interview with former SSA official involved in legislation.

121. Senate Report 92–1230, pp. 289–91.

122. Interviews with present and former officials in BHI's Division of State Operations.

123. Interview with involved BHI official.

Professional Peer Review: SSA and the Practice of Medicine

Most of the Medicare law's requirements for hospital quality reflected existing hospital practice. But there was one exception: the requirement that each hospital establish a committee of physicians to review and evaluate their use of the hospital. This "utilization review committee" was to review the admissions, length of stay, and professional services for Medicare beneficiaries, and to determine the "medical necessity" of any beneficiary's stay of "extended duration." If the committee found that a continued stay in the hospital was not "medically necessary," Medicare payments would cease three days later.[1]

Physicians had been reviewing the quality of each others' practices before Medicare. Tissue committees that reviewed the practice of surgery, for example, had existed and been required for JCAH accreditation for several years.[2] But peer review directed toward efficient use of hospital resources was much less established.[3] Its objective was to have physicians use the hospital as much as necessary and no more, and it involved a review of both the cost and quality of hospital care.

Although using the hospital too little can be as harmful to patients as using it too much, utilization review has focused primarily on preventing unnecessary hospitalization.

Excessive use is also justifiably interpreted as poor quality, and for several reasons. Procedures performed may be inappropriate and potentially harmful, even though actual harm to the patient may occur infrequently. This is certainly true for unnecessary surgery, since any surgery always carries some risk, no matter how small. It is also true for unnecessary hospitalization, since all hospitalization implies some risk of hospital-acquired infection, atrophy of disuse and trauma, as well as social and psychological damage.[4]

Utilization review was to prevent such consequences by increasing physicians' awareness of the most effective and least costly ways to treat patients.

The cost more than the quality implications of unnecessary hospitalization explains why it received so much attention. Studies of hospital use around the country revealed substantial variation in length of stay.[5] In 1965 an AMA official explained to his peers what these variations could mean in dollars:

The hospital, providing the tools used by the physician in giving necessary care for his patients, is itself an expensive tool. The cost per patient day in the average short-term general hospital was $41.58 last year—again the mythical average. The cost of this tool in some instances runs as high as $80 per day. As physicians are mainly responsible for calling this tool into play, it should be their responsibility to use it with a high degree of sophistication.[6]

Because of the cost implications of hospital use, the Medicare law did not leave physicians to undertake this responsibility voluntarily. The utilization review requirement made it government's job to see that care was reviewed. In the absence of professionally initiated review processes, Medicare administrators had to decide how much to require of the medical profession and how to enforce whatever they required.

If SSA had followed a cost-effectiveness strategy, officials would have approached this task by developing measures of desirable or efficient hospital use. Hospitals and their medical staffs would have to conform to these measures as a condition for participation in Medicare. Alternatively, with a balancing strategy, SSA would have assessed competing interests on utilization review and made their policy a compromise. In fact, SSA took a middle road between exercising and abdicating government authority over hospitals and physicians. Despite AMA pressure, SSA refused to ignore the cost control aspects of utilization review, but in developing specific review requirements and in monitoring compliance with them, SSA's strategy was to interfere as little as possible with the medical profession.

Defining Utilization Review

The law mandated two types of review by utilization review committees: (1) general reviews of patterns of practice and (2) specific reviews of cases of long stays. Organized medicine viewed the first as a legitimate educational activity for the medical staff, but they opposed the second as an unacceptable "policing" role.[7] A former hospital association lobbyist described the AMA's position:[8] Having decided to encourage physicians to cooperate with the law, the AMA then asked "How do we protect ourselves?" The answer, according to this participant, was to make certain that Medicare would treat utilization review as an "educational" mechanism rather than a device for fiscal control.

When SSA consulted industry representatives on utilization review, the AMA pressed this position. Arguing that utilization review should be primarily an educational rather than a policing device, an AMA spokesman proposed that it focus on statistical reviews rather than reviews of individual cases.[9]

This position contradicted the law's requirements and the congressional intent behind them. In its report on the Medicare law, The Senate Finance Committee explained that it was

particularly concerned that the utilization and review function is carried out in a manner which protects the patients while at the same time making certain that they remain in the hospital only so long as is necessary, and that every effort be made to move them from the hospital to other facilities which can provide less expensive, but equal, care to meet their current medical needs.[10]

Perhaps for this reason, program administrators would not accede to the physicians' request. Both Public Health Service (PHS) and Bureau of Health Insurance (BHI) officials explained to physician consultants that case review was part of the law and that the program would have to recognize the "control aspects" of utilization review.[11]

In developing the specifics of control, however, SSA was much more willing to leave the profession on its own. First of all, SSA never used its authority to specify what constituted a long stay.[12] The law had anticipated that this would be done in regulations, for which the committees suggested some guidelines:

Regulations would provide the institution some leeway in determining when the review would have to be carried out, and the point at which a review would be most appropriate might vary with the diagnosis and treatment involved.[13]

But SSA did not define long stays by diagnosis or any other way. Based on the "preponderant opinion" of their consultants, SSA left the definition of extended stay to each individual hospital and its medical staff.[14]

A second decision on control involved a review committee's finding that continued care was not medically necessary. In their first draft of regulations, SSA proposed that Medicare coverage be cut off only when such findings were unanimous. The Health Insurance Benefits Advisory Council (HIBAC), apparently more willing as professionals to make demands on their peers, rejected this proposal and the agency withdrew it.[15]

On a third issue, SSA and HIBAC cooperated to avoid imposing external authority on hospitals and physicians. Arthur Hess, then BHI director, consulted HIBAC on utilization review requirements for hospitals in which staff doctors had a financial interest.[16] Presumably this was a problem because physician owners make money from keeping people in the hospital and therefore are unable to review hospital use objectively. In addressing this problem, both BHI and HIBAC members showed far more concern for institutional independence than for eliminating conflicts of interest. Hess informed the Council that if doctors with a financial interest were excluded from utilization review committees, many small hospitals would find it difficult to establish a committee without the aid of local medical societies or public health organizations.[17] The Medicare law offered some guidance on this question by specifying what to do where

. . . because of the small size of the institution . . . or for such other reason or reasons as may be included in regulations, it is impractical for the institution to have a properly functioning staff committee. . . .[18]

In such cases, the law required that review be performed by

a group outside the institution . . . which is established by the local medical society and some or all of the hospitals and extended care facilities in the locality, or . . . which is established in such other manner as may be approved by the Secretary.[19]

Neither officials nor Council members even mentioned this requirement in their discussion. Instead HIBAC

concluded that the real need was not to exclude physicians with a financial interest but to assure the inclusion of physicians *without* a financial interest. The Council agreed that the utilization review committee should be required to include at least one member who does not have a financial interest in the hospital.[20]

How this might prevent conflict of interest was not recorded.

When it came to general patterns of hospital care, SSA showed little interest in guiding hospitals' review activity. Although the agency observed in 1966 that the review process could be encouraged by compiling data "which would permit each provider to compare its utilization experience with that of comparable providers on a local, regional and national basis,"[21] they were slow to follow through. In 1970 the staff of the Senate Finance Committee reported:

In the early stages of the program, the Social Security Administration discouraged the intermediaries from collecting such data and furnishing it to the institutions on a regular basis for their use. It indicated that it would be developing such data on a detailed and comprehensive basis and would send the data directly to hospitals and extended care facilities. Unfortunately, the Social Security Administration did not live up to its promises. After more than three years of experience under the program the Social Security Administration is just now completing a sample study of utilization of services *in one state*.[22]

SSA's Office of Research and Statistics (ORS) finally developed a data system in 1969 and made it available to hospitals in 1970. But, according to officials, institutions found fault with the system and did not use it, and BHI showed no interest in imposing it on them.[23]

Enforcing Utilization Review

The Medicare law charged SSA with more than deciding what hospitals should be doing in utilization review. SSA also had to decide how to monitor what hospitals actually *were* doing. The law allowed the secretary to delegate responsbility for overseeing utilization review to one or both of two administrative agents: the state health agencies, who were generally responsible for evaluating hospital compliance with Medicare's quality requirements, and the fiscal agents or intermediaries whose primary job was making payments. Choosing between these agents had important implications for both the nature and enforcement of utilization review. If SSA decided to rely primarily on state agencies, Medicare would evaluate utilization review along with all its other requirements for hospital quality. A hospital that failed to meet utilization review requirements would be denied participation in the program. Relying on intermediaries, on the other hand, meant overseeing utilization review as part of the payment process and did not entail an enforcement mechanism. Intermediaries were private insurers, primarily Blue Cross plans. As they reviewed claims to determine whether to pay for services received, some of these plans reviewed appropriateness of admission, length of stay, and services rendered.[24] While "claims review" can involve questions and data similar to those appropriate for utilization review, by itself it is neither a review of patterns of practice nor a review concurrent with a stay in the hospital.

Although both agents could play a role in utilization review, distribution of authority between them influenced whether review of hospital use would focus primarily on quality enforcement or on benefit payment. By relying primarily on intermediaries, SSA opted for the latter and minimized its responsibility for what went on inside the hospital. Congressional testimony, advisory consultations, and policy outcomes reveal the political and administrative advantages of this choice.

Medicare strategists developed the concept of "fiscal intermediary" in 1962 in order to win support for Medicare from the then-waivering American Hospital Association (AHA). Because the AHA was affiliated with Blue Cross,[25] Medicare proposals had always specified that hospitals could use Blue Cross plans to represent them in negotiating terms of participation in a government insurance program. In 1962, the Blue Cross role was expanded by allowing the organization nominated by a hospital to determine payments on the hospital's behalf, subject to review by the secretary, and to perform various consultative services, among them assistance in utilization review.[26] This provision was in the final legislation.[27] A former hospital association lobbyist said it was the AHA who "sold" Wilbur Cohen on the use of Blue Cross as a buffer between the hospitals and government.[28] As HEW explained to the Senate Finance Committee in 1965, this "buffer between the hospital and the federal government," would enable Medicare (and apparently the hospitals) "to benefit . . . from the relationships [the intermediaries] have established with hospitals, physicians, and others who furnish health care."[29]

Congress heard testimony on the use of this buffer, rather than a government agency, to oversee utilization review. The American Hospital Association strongly opposed government (state agency) involvement in utilization review and hospital payment. Walter McNerney, president of the Blue Cross Association, which ultimately became the intermediary for most of the nation's hospitals, supported and explained the hospitals' point of view. He observed that hospitals were afraid that state oversight implied government involvement in the practice of medicine. Delegating oversight to intermediaries, he argued, would create less of a confrontation.[30]

For precisely that reason, labor spokesmen told Congress not to grant intermediaries responsibility for oversight. Mel Glasser of the United Auto Workers questioned whether the public could expect an arms-length review of hospital operations from organizations which had initially been included in the program to represent hospitals.[31]

Wilbur Mills, then chairman of the House Ways and Means Committee, summarized the question that Congress had to face:

How do we get the most out of such a utilization review plan and the least criticism of our use of it? Do we get less criticism of our use of it, essential as we think it is, if we call upon some agent outside of Government to see to it that it is performed, carried out, or if we try to do it ourselves directly through an agency of the Government?[32]

Rather than answer this question, Congress left the decision to administrative discretion.[33]

When SSA discussed the matter with industry consultants, physicians reiterated their fear that utilization review could lead to government control over the practice of medicine. They recommended that state agencies be prohibited from case reviews and ongoing evaluation of utilization review, and that their role be limited to assessment of written review plans.[34] Neither SSA nor HIBAC would go this far in limiting state agency responsibility, but they responded to physician concerns by giving intermediaries primary responsibility for overseeing review.

In November 1965, BHI Director Hess told HIBAC of a "public relations problem" on utilization review. BHI's initial guidelines and reports of "staffing-up" of some state agencies had contributed, he said, to growing apprehension by physicians and hospital administrators that state agencies would exercise unwarranted supervision over review activities. In response to this concern Hess observed that, under the law, state agencies would investigate whether a satisfactory utilization review plan had been established and make recommendations, but that intermediaries would carry on much of the ongoing oversight activities. HIBAC concurred in this decision.[35]

As intermediaries and state agencies pressed BHI to clarify their responsibility, the agency elaborated its policy in a memorandum.[36] The memorandum emphasized that state agencies would have "sole responsibility" for assessing institutional compliance with Medicare certification requirements. But at the same time, those requirements were significantly circumscribed. Initially, state agencies were to focus on written descriptions of utilization review plans. State agencies were to consult with the provider about any defects and to assist in establishing a satisfactory plan *at the provider's request*. Although state agencies were authorized to review data and to conduct studies, including on-site reviews, to determine compliance, primary responsibility for evaluating and improving ongoing utilization review was specifically delegated to intermediaries.[37] Furthermore, a later memorandum indicated that in on-site and other reviews, determinations of compliance were restricted to conformity of actual review activities to the written plan and to the procedural requirements of the regulations.[38]

BHI distinguished between procedure and performance in outlining intermediary responsibilities.

A provider may, for example, have a properly constituted committee which performs the necessary services, completes work sheets, keeps minutes, prepares charts and reports, etc., but the facility may not actually be taking meaningful steps to analyze and follow through on the information that is produced as a result of the activity.[39]

The latter was a matter for intermediary assistance and encouragement,[40] not state agency enforcement.

Having state agencies look at procedure rather than performance was consistent with other standard-setting practices. As chapter 2 describes, JCAH and then Medicare looked primarily at structure rather than performance in reviewing hospital quality. But in this particular case, performance was explicitly recognized and separated from enforcement.

Documents and interviews provide several explanations for BHI's decision to give intermediaries primary responsibility for overseeing review. BHI officials justified it in terms of "operational logic." Intermediaries, they felt, had direct daily contact with hospitals because of their payment responsibility. In reviewing claims for payment, they would see data on hospital use that would enable them to evaluate and advise the utilization review committee. Furthermore, intermediaries had a financial interest in monitoring utilization for their private beneficiaries. State agencies, on the other hand, had demonstrated neither ability nor interest in overseeing hospitals. In both experience and interest, BHI officials believed intermediaries would surpass state agencies as monitors of effective utilization review.[41]

A PHS official offered further explanation for BHI's decision. BHI was inappropriately associating utilization review with claims review, this official said, and treating it as a determination of coverage according to rules for payment instead of a qualitative evaluation of medical care.[42] Thus SSA emphasized the job of the payment agent and failed to encourage state agencies to measure and evaluate professional performance.

Different SSA and PHS persepctives correspond to differences in the agencies' experience and perceptions of themselves. PHS comprised public health officials who frequently had worked or would work in state agencies. Further-more, PHS was responsible for relations with state agencies in Medicare and other federal health programs. Thus for both professional and bureaucratic reasons, they believed that utilization review was a qualitative evaluation of medical care that should be reviewed by health professionals in the state agencies. Medicare officials in SSA, on the other hand, were experienced in social insurance pro-grams. Like Blue Cross personnel, they were familiar with evaluating claims for appropriate payment. Thus they had a bias toward claims review and an affinity with intermediaries.

These explanations suggest that BHI was not conscientiously avoiding antagonizing hospitals and physicians, but rather wanted to avoid the com-plexities of quality review, with which they were unfamiliar. BHI officials them-selves acknowledge that they did not understand utilization review in the begin-ning, and point out that it was poorly understood in the field by both inter-mediaries and state agencies. Policies were guidelines more than a rigid division of labor, said one official, and "flexibility" in regulation was the general rule.[43] No matter how difficult the situation, however, SSA's focus on administrative convenience was remarkably single-minded. Totally absent from their policy deliberations was an assessment of the enforcement implications of their choice of administrative agents. The lineup of political interests behind the alternatives suggests that this gap was as much a product of SSA's political as administrative interests in avoiding conflict with hospitals and physicians. Achievement of the hospital industry's cooperation was the fundamental, if unarticulated, premise on which utilization review's implementation, like the legislation behind it, was based.

Evidence on actual compliance with procedural requirements for utilization review further demonstrates SSA reluctance to make requirements of hospitals. Of a sample of hospitals reviewed in mid-1968, SSA found that 10 percent did not review long-stay cases; 47 percent did not review admissions; and 42 percent did not maintain abstracts of medical records or other summary forms for evaluating services.[44] Reviews of certification suggest that state agency reluctance to become involved in utilization review had much to do with the record of non-compliance.[45] But, as with certification in general, this reluctance was reinforced by SSA's educational approach. Describing the agency's extensive effort to edu-cate people in the field on utilization review, a BHI official asked rhetorically: "Do you kick a hospital out of the program if it is giving good care but does poor utilization review?"[46] Apparently not, even though it was a statutory requirement for participation. Threatened with termination, another official explained, a hospital could always promise to cooperate and to comply "from now on."[47] Given the agency's consultative approach to certification and the limited nature of its utilization review requirements, such a promise prevented termination.[48]

Termination was not, however, the only sanction available to SSA for enforcing utilization review. In hospitals that failed to make "timely review" of long stays, the secretary could limit Medicare coverage to twenty days.[49] Such an action required advance notice to both the hospital and the public. SSA never used this "twenty day rule." While some officials attributed this to administrative complications or the arbitrary nature of the rule, others indicated that a penalty for inadequate utilization review was simply considered inappropriate. As with termination, said one official, a hospital could simply avoid the sanction by promising to do better. "So," he asked, "why bother?"[50]

The staff of the Senate Finance Committee summarized the consequences of this policy in 1970:

. . . the utilization review requirements have, generally speaking, been of a token nature and ineffective as a curb to unnecessary use of institutional care and services. Utilization review in Medicare can be characterized as more form than substance.[51]

Maintaining Noninterference

Limited enforcement of utilization review continued to appeal to SSA both administratively and politically, but its ineffectiveness soon created pressure for a reassessment. The problem arose with skilled nursing homes, then called extended care facilities (ECFs). Congress included ECFs in Medicare so that beneficiaries could receive skilled nursing care in a setting less expensive than a hospital. But they did not intend to cover the nonmedical or custodial care that these institutions might also provide. As claims for ECF benefits began to come in, it became apparent that beneficiaries and institutions were not observing this distinction. Program costs were consequently far higher than anticipated.[52]

Unlike quality, costs were a major concern to SSA. As a review of their payment policy will show,[53] officials preferred to avoid cost increases that necessitated tax increases. In this case, there were two ways administrators could try to curtail excessive costs. They could enforce utilization review, which was intended to ensure that only "medically necessary" services were covered, or they could ignore utilization review committee decisions and allow intermediaries to control claims payment independently. SSA had already avoided enforcing utilization review, equated utilization review with claims review, and relied heavily on intermediaries. Authorizing intermediaries to deny inappropriate claims was the next logical step. Claims denial rather than enforcement of utilization review was SSA's response to unnecessary or uncovered care. Denial of payment did not prevent charges that SSA was interfering in the practice of medicine. But by focusing on appropriate payment rather than medical necessity, SSA avoided direct decisions about professional practice.

After some equivocation at the start of Medicare,[54] SSA ruled that a utilization review committee's finding on medical necessity was the conclusive determinant of an individual's right to Medicare benefits, not subject to rebuttal or reversal by SSA.[55] In discussing this decision, a HIBAC member asked whether someone could appeal a committee finding on grounds that the committee had not followed prescribed procedures. Mel Blumenthal of HEW's general counsel's office replied that "such a contention would not seem to affect the determination made in the individual case—that, for the purpose of determining the right of the individual to hospital insurance benefits, the Administration (SSA) was bound under the statute by the decision of the utilization review committee." He also said that to interpret the law otherwise "would undermine the authority of utilization review committees to a point where they would become ineffective."[56]

Although legal counsel maintained this position, SSA did not.[57] In response to excessive ECF claims, they decided that utilization review committee decisions on "medical necessity" were no longer binding, and that intermediaries should make independent determinations of program coverage. Arguing that there was a difference between medical and coverage decisions, BHI explained to HIBAC

. . . that if the intermediary were not permitted to question and where appropriate disallow a request for payment which involved noncovered care simply because of the existence of a physician's certification or a utilization review committee's finding with respect to the need for institutionalization, the program would be paying for care which the law specifically excluded from coverage. Since the financing of the program did not contemplate payment for such care, the financial status of the program would be adversely affected.[58]

To reinforce their case, BHI argued that allowing intermediaries to disregard utilization review committee decisions would enhance procedural as well as substantive compliance with the law. BHI enumerated potential procedural mistakes that committees might make: determining retroactively that a stay was not medically necessary; failing to take into account availability and appropriateness of alternative facilities; failing to give proper notice of their decision to affected parties; and failure to consult with attending physicians or to give weight to their decisions. If an intermediary found such defects, BHI explained, all it could do under the old policy was to bring them to the attention of the committee and suggest that they be corrected. If the committee did not change its ways, "the intermediary could, presumably," call the matter to the attention of the state agency. If the intermediary had ·independent payment authority, on the other hand, it could "approve, deny, or adjust payment as it determined appropriate and consistent with the law."[59]

Despite concern that this would "undercut" rather than reinforce utilization review, as this statement implied, HIBAC endorsed[60] and BHI promulgated the intermediaries' new authority.[61] The record shows no consideration of the alternative way to control institutional use, that is, having state agencies enforce compliance with desired guidelines for utilization review.

Although large scale denial of claims changed the care provided to Medicare beneficiaries,[62] it did so by ignoring utilization review rather than enforcing it.

Claims review could not prevent retroactive determination that care was unnecessary, a goal that BHI mentioned. It was itself a determination of coverage after care had been received. Sylvia Law and the Health Law Project of the University of Pennsylvania described in detail what this difference can mean to beneficiaries. The Medicare law's utilization review requirements, if enforced,

assured that the individual would always have timely notice before Medicare payments were terminated on the grounds that services were not medically necessary. If the provider was an approved participating institution, the individual could safely assume that it had an adequate utilization review committee and that committee would give him timely notice if it made an adverse determination of the medical necessity of continued treatment. If the provider was under a twenty day order, the individual would know, before he or she entered the institution, that care beyond the twentieth day might not be paid for and could make plans depending upon the anticipated length of stay and the availability of alternative institutions.[63]

Retroactive denial of coverage has none of these safeguards. It leaves the individual financially liable for care he or she has already received. Recognizing this fact, institutions can deny service to beneficiaries who cannot guarantee they will be able to pay. If this occurs, beneficiaries have no recourse.[64]

Several years after this change in policy, rising Medicare costs again raised the issue of effective utilization review. Although BHI made some new proposals of its own, the impetus for change came primarily from Congress. While sensitive to the need for fiscal control, SSA opposed changes that increased government responsibility for overseeing professional practice and preferred to rely on control of benefit payments.

In 1969 and 1970 proposals for peer review of medical care appeared frequently in discussions of rapidly rising medical costs.[65] Reflecting quality as well as cost concerns, in 1969 HIBAC recommended legislation that would authorize the secretary to make quality requirements of physicians and to discontinue Medicare payments to physicians and suppliers on evidence of fraud, repeated overcharging, or excessive or harmful services.[66] HEW then introduced an amendment on termination for abuse, which proposed establishing "program review teams" to review individual cases and overall utilization data. These teams would consist of physicians, other professional personnel in the health field, and consumer representatives, but only the professional members of the team would participate in case reviews involving "excessive, inferior or harmful services." Primarily a means of preventing what officials called "bad actors" from participating in Medicare, the new review mechanism was "not intended to supplant existing peer review structures, but rather to complement and enhance present arrangements."[67]

At about the same time, the AMA developed a peer review proposal of its own and asked Senator Wallace Bennett (R-Utah) to introduce it.[68] They proposed to have state medical societies establish Peer Review Organizations to review allegations of overcharging or questionable practices in Medicare or other federal programs, and to recommend disciplinary action to the secretary of HEW.[69]

Rather than support this proposal, as the AMA had anticipated, Senator Bennett developed his own peer review program that went far beyond either of the above. He proposed the establishment of Professional Standards Review Organizations (PSROs) to review both the care provided by individual practitioners and overall utilization data, and to develop and apply norms for care and treatment. In designating PSROs, HEW was to give priority to local medical societies; but where they proved unable or unwilling to do the job, HEW could contract with state or local health departments or other organizations.[70]

The PSRO proposal was a direct response to the Senate Finance Committee's finding "that the present system of assuring proper utilization of institutional and physicians' services is basically inadequate."[71] The committee also recognized physician "resentment that their medical determinations are challenged by insurance company personnel." Their solution was to restructure the review process, make it fully responsible for Medicare coverage decisions, and increase its effectiveness "through substantially increased professional participation." At the same time,

the committee does not intend any abdication of public responsibility or accountability in recommending the professional standards review organizations approach. While persuaded that comprehensive review through a unified mechanism is necessary and that it should be done through usage, wherever possible and wherever feasible, of medical organizations, the committee would not preclude other arrangements being made by the Secretary where medical organizations are unwilling or unable to assume the required work or where such organizations function not as an effective professional effort to assure proper utilization and quality of care but rather as a token buffer designed to create an illusion of professional concern.[72]

The objective was to establish a review process run by physicians but accountable to government, to control Medicare services by influencing medical practice.

PSROs differed from utilization review committees primarily because they were independent of hospitals. But authority to pursue the Finance Committee's objective was in the law all along. SSA had simply not used it. It is therefore not surprising that they opposed the introduction of the system they had managed to avoid.

BHI officials' reactions to the PSRO proposal show their commitment to existing administrative procedures and their reluctance to depend on physicians for control over coverage. A former official described his agency as "horrified" at the prospect of total disruption of their review and payment system and the establishment of a whole new apparatus. If the objective was to give physicians greater responsibility in the review of services, explained one official, physicians could review the claims data collected by fiscal agents. But to establish an entirely new review system and place it in the middle of the payment process was an expensive exercise in "empire-building." BHI officials agreed that utilization review was a failure, but they felt they had greater control over their program through intermediaries than they would through PSROs.[73]

BHI's views had little impact on the PSRO legislation. Although enthusiasm for PSROs was less than wholehearted in the rest of HEW, the department's official position was to support Senator Bennett. The senator had loyally supported the Nixon administration's proposal for national health insurance. As the ranking Republican member of the Senate Finance Committee, Bennett deserved a favor in return, observed one participant. Furthermore, a new idea had some appeal to a department scrambling for a solution to a "health care crisis" they had proclaimed.[74] The PSRO proposal became law in late 1972.[75] Partly because SSA had opposed its enactment, authority for PSRO implementation was delegated to the assistant secretary for health rather than to SSA.[76]

Conclusion

SSA's failure to develop and enforce standards for utilization review is consistent with its balancing strategy on quality enforcement. With little to gain and much to lose from antagonizing hospitals and physicians, administrators preferred not to evaluate what went on inside the hospital. Interviews did not reveal concern about challenging the medical profession directly behind every decision, but this concern shaped the context in which decisions were made, and the results served that purpose.

This balancing strategy was reinforced by SSA's inclination to do what came most easily to it. Officials were experienced in paying benefits, not delivering medical care, and they approached the review process accordingly. By defining utilization review as a question of payment and relying on an administrative apparatus that sidestepped enforcement, SSA could avoid involvement in the practice of medicine. This approach had the additional advantage of controlling costs without controlling physicians or institutions. In sum, what was administratively complicated in utilization review was also politically controversial. SSA's strategy was to avoid both.

Notes

1. 42 U.S.C. sec. 1395f(a) and sec. 1395x(k).

2. Feather Davis Hair, "Hospital Accreditation: A Developmental Study of the Social Control of Institutions" (Ph.D. dissertation, Vanderbilt University, 1972), pp. 171 ff.

3. For development of utilization review, see Nancy C. Maki, Daniel Walden, and Lawrence Cohen, "Medicare's Effects on Medical Care: Issues and

Outlook," *Public Health Reports* 83 (September 1968): 708–13; and presentations to AMA Utilization Review Conference, *Journal of the American Medical Association* 196 (June 13, 1966): 994–1009.

4. Avedis Donabedian, *A Guide to Medical Care Administration*, Vol. 2 (New York: American Public Health Association, 1969), pp. 11–12.

5. See, for example, John M. Rumsey, "Utilization Review Committees: Statement of the Problem," *Journal of the American Medical Association* 196 (June 13, 1966): 994–5.

6. Ibid., p. 994, reprinted with permission.

7. Ibid., p. 995.

8. Interview. The American Hospital Association, composed of hospital administrators, seemed to disagree with the AMA, perceiving utilization review as a contribution to cost control and, presumably, control over hospitals' medical staffs. See comments from AHA spokesman, HIBAC materials, Consultant Work Groups, Subcommittee on Utilization Review of Work Group on Physician Participation, summary of meeting, November 5, 1965, pp. 2–3 (hereafter cited as Subcommittee on Utilization Review).

9. Ibid.

10. Excerpts from Report of Committee on Finance, U.S. Senate, to Accompany H.R. 6675, 1965, p. 47 in New Members Background Book, Part I, for Health Insurance Benefits Advisory Council (HIBAC), 1968.

11. Subcommittee on Utilization Review, pp. 2, 3, and 5.

12. See critique of utilization review under Medicare in U.S., Congress, Senate, Committee on Finance, *Medicare and Medicaid: Problems, Issues and Alternatives*, Report of the Staff to the Senate Finance Committee, 91st Cong., 1st sess., February 9, 1970, pp. 105–9 (hereafter cited as *Medicare and Medicaid* report).

13. Excerpts from Report of the Committee on Finance, U.S. Senate, to Accompany H.R. 6675, p. 47; and from Report of the Committee on Ways and Means on H.R. 6675, House of Representatives, p. 41; both in *New Members Background Book*, Part I, HIBAC, 1968.

14. Arthur E. Hess, "Medicare and Utilization Review," *Journal of the American Medical Association* 196 (June 13, 1966): 996 and 997.

15. HIBAC minutes, II, November 21, 1965, p. 7.

16. Ibid., p. 10.

17. Ibid., p. 10.

18. 42 U.S.C. sec. 1395x(k).

19. 42 U.S.C. sec. 1395x(k) (2).

20. HIBAC minutes, II, November 21, 1965, p. 10. Emphasis in original.

21. "Responsibilities of Intermediaries and State Agencies in the Area of Provider Utilization Practices," Staff Memorandum for HIBAC, HIBAC Agenda Book, April 30–May 1, 1966, p. 3.

22. *Medicare and Medicaid* report, p. 109. Emphasis in original.

23. Discussion of Medicare Analysis of Days of Care (MADOC) with officials in the Office of Research and Statistics and a former BHI official. For a more detailed review of MADOC with similar conclusions, see Diane Rowland, "Data Rich and Information Poor: Medicare's Resources for Prospective Rate Setting," Harvard University Center for Community Health and Medical Care, Report Series R-45-12 July 1976, pp. 36-9.

24. For a discussion of Blue Cross review activities, see James M. Ensign (Director of Professional Relations, Blue Cross Association), "Third-Party Review Programs from the Blue Cross Vantage Point," *Journal of the American Medical Association* 196 (June 13, 1966): 1006-7.

25. Blue Cross was created by hospitals and the AHA, and until 1972 the name "Blue Cross" and the Blue Cross insignia were owned by the AHA. For an informative account of Blue Cross, both in itself and as part of Medicare administration, see Sylvia Law, *Blue Cross: What Went Wrong?*, prepared by the Health Law Project, University of Pennsylvania (New Haven: Yale University Press, 1974).

26. For legislative history and explanation of the change, see "Health Insurance for Aged Persons," July 24, 1961, in U.S. Department of Health, Education, and Welfare, Social Security Administration, *Background on Medicare 1957-1962; Reports, Studies and Congressional Considerations on Health Legislation*, 2 vols., 85th-87th Congress, pp. 76-77 and legislative proposals included therein; Peter A. Corning, *The Evolution of Medicare . . . from Idea to Law*, Department of Health, Education, and Welfare, Social Security Administration, Office of Research and Statistics, Research Report no. 29, p. 92 and n. 22, and p. 98, n. 26; and Law, *Blue Cross*, pp. 32-33 and n. 188. The interpretation on page 32 of the AHA resolution quoted in n. 188 is somewhat misleading. Law also discusses an HEW memorandum on this subject and administrative considerations on the use of Blue Cross, pp. 34-41.

27. 42 U.S.C. sec. 1395h(b).

28. Interview. Blue Cross, he said, had objections to being both a hospital and a government agent. "We forced it on them," he recalled.

29. U.S., Congress, Senate, Committee on Finance, *Hearings on H.R. 6675*, 89th Cong., 1st sess., p. 202 and pp. 204-6.

30. U.S., Congress, House, Committee on Ways and Means, *Medical Care for the Aged: Executive Hearings on H.R. 1 and Other Proposals for Medical Care for the Aged*, 89th Cong., 1st sess., 1965, p. 173, pp. 176-77, p. 228, and pp. 287-89. Although McNerney said "carriers," his comment applied generally to fiscal agents.

31. Ibid., pp. 490-95. The Teamsters also opposed the Blue Cross role. See Senate Finance Committee, *Hearings on H.R. 6675*, 1965, p. 272, and UAW testimony, pp. 1252-53. Testimony dealt with intermediary responsibility for both fiscal and quality issues, but the former was more readily accepted than the latter.

32. Committee on Ways and Means, *Medical Care for the Aged*, 1965, p. 203.

33. Excerpts from Ways and Means Committee, Reports to Accompany H.R. 6675, p. 44; Finance, p. 51.

34. Consultant Work Groups, summary of meeting, November 19, 1965, pp. 2-3. On the issue, the AMA and the AHA were in agreement.

35. HIBAC minutes, II, November 21, 1965, pp. 7-10. On the request of the physicians work group, Hess presented their recommendation that state agencies be prohibited from case reviews and ongoing evaluation of utilization review, limiting their role to assessing the adequacy of plans submitted to them. HIBAC did not prohibit state agency review, but recommended that state agencies "concentrate first on the initial job of certification and then work out procedures for ongoing evaluation with the intermediaries and carriers . . . in consultation with appropriate professional organizations and consumer groups." (This was one of the few references to consumers in the HIBAC minutes from 1965 through 1971.) At the consultant work group meeting three weeks later, Hess explained that state agencies could not be prohibited from involvement in utilization review but that guidelines had been revised and the major assignment in this area would be given to fiscal intermediaries. The state agencies would supplement the assistance offered to providers by hospital associations and intermediaries. Consultant work groups, summary of meeting, December 10, 1965.

36. "Responsibilities of Intermediaries and State Agencies in the Area of Provider Utilization Practices," Staff Memorandum for HIBAC, HIBAC Agenda Book, April 30-May 1, 1966, p. 1.

37. Ibid., pp. 1-2. Reliance on a state agency, however, was not ruled out if it were the local choice, apparently of the intermediary and the state agency. Communication between intermediaries and state agencies was also expected.

38. "Role of Intermediaries and State Agencies in Utilization Review," staff memorandum prepared for HIBAC, appendix A to HIBAC minutes, XVI, June 3-4, 1967, p. 5.

39. Ibid., p. 2.

40. Ibid.

41. Interviews with present and former BHI and HEW officials, and HIBAC, "Responsibilities of Intermediaries and State Agencies in the Area of Provider Utilization Practices," p. 2. One former HEW official suggested that the administrative choice was between two unsatisfactory alternatives.

42. Interview with former PHS official. This issue was the subject of conflict between BHI and PHS. A former PHS official recalled that BHI wanted to eliminate the state agency role altogether but bowed to pressure from PHS. Other interviews suggest that there was also conflict on the subject between the Divisions of State Operations and Contract Operations within BHI.

43. Interviews with BHI officials. See also comments on flexibility for providers and their medical staffs in HIBAC, "Role of Intermediaries and State Agencies in Utilization Review," 1967 memo, p. 1.

44. *Medicare and Medicaid* report, p. 107.

45. "Summary of Program Review Findings and State Agency Recommendations," Staff Report for Subcommittee on Hospital and Extended Care Services, Committee on the Evaluation of Delivery and Utilization of Services (CEDUS), HIBAC, p. 4; and discussions of utilization review in Selected State Reports; both in HIBAC, Task Force on Hospital and Extended Care Services, Notebook, September 9-12, 1968. A preliminary draft of HIBAC's first annual report was critical of SSA's enforcement of utilization review. "Utilization Review," Report of Task Force on Hospital and Extended Care Services, CEDUS Agenda Book, December 30, 1968, pp. 1-2.

46. Interview with official in BHI's Division of State Operations.

47. Interview with official in BHI's Division of State Operations.

48. BHI data on terminations indicate failure to undertake utilization review as the reason for termination in one case. Law, *Blue Cross*, n. 669, cites a BHI official's argument that hospitals with utilization review deficiencies usually had other serious deficiencies leading to termination as the reason that unsatisfactory utilization review was not the reason for termination. But the evidence cited above challenges this assertion.

49. 42 U.S.C. sec. 1395cc(d).

50. Interviews with present and former BHI and PHS officials.

51. *Medicare and Medicaid* report, p. 105.

52. For discussion of this problem, see Law, *Blue Cross*, Chapter 5, and HIBAC minutes, XVI:2, June 4, 1967, Tucker's explanation, p. 20.

53. See chapter 4.

54. Consultant Work Group. Subcommittee on Utilization Review of Work Group on Physician Participation, November 5, 1965, pp. 4-5. Interestingly, an AMA representative felt "very strongly that without a direct cost control, i.e., a claims review by the fiscal intermediary with clear-cut guidelines for refusing payment for clearly unwarranted services, utilization review will be a waste of time." Tucker of BHI indicated that they had not yet decided whether to adopt a "hard" or "soft" position, with independent intermediary authority considered the former. The April 1966 memo on intermediary-state agency responsibilities was the first indication that SSA had rejected this approach. HIBAC, "Responsibilities of Intermediaries and State Agencies in the Area of Provider Utilization Practices," p. 4.

55. Discussed in HIBAC minutes, XI:1, September 10, 1966, pp. 17-18. The issue arose with respect to another provision in the law—the relationship between the utilization review committee decision and the attending physician—but the principle discussed was more broadly applicable.

56. Ibid. Blumenthal qualified his comments with the observation that his office had not yet studied the case in question.

57. HIBAC minutes, XVI: 2, June 4, 1967, pp. 21–22.

58. "The Role of Fiscal Intermediaries in Claims Review," Staff Memorandum for HIBAC, in HIBAC Agenda Book, June 3–4, 1967, and HIBAC minutes, VI:2, June 4, 1967, pp. 20–22.

59. HIBAC, "The Role of Fiscal Intermediaries in Claims Review."

60. HIBAC minutes, XVI:2, June 4, 1967, pp. 21–22.

61. See Law, *Blue Cross*, p. 122 and n. 671. Law argues that BHI did not have statutory authority for this action. On legislative history, see especially p. 121, with accompanying citations. BHI sent instructions to intermediaries, August 14, 1967, in BHI Intermediary Letter 257, printed in U.S., Congress, Senate, Committee on Finance, *Hearings before Senate Finance Committee on H.R. 12080*, 90th Cong., 1st sess., 1967, p. 1042.

62. The impact of claims denial was primarily on Extended Care Facilities, many of which dropped out of Medicare as a result. See Law, *Blue Cross*, pp. 123–25, notes 676–79.

63. Ibid., p. 120.

64. Ibid., pp. 123–25. Law reports elsewhere that HEW did try to deal with this problem with an Assurance of Payment procedure introduced in 1968, p. 138, nn. 768, 769. Only ECFs with functioning utilization review committees, she states, could take advantage of the procedure. The 1972 Social Security amendments prohibited retroactive claim denial where the beneficiary and provider acted in good faith. P.L. 92–603, sec. 1879. For this and related changes in the law, see Law, *Blue Cross*, pp. 130–135.

65. See, for example, "The Nation's Health Care System," Remarks of the President, HEW Secretary Robert A. Finch, Assistant Secretary Roger L. Egeberg and Undersecretary John G. Veneman on a Report on Health Care Problems and Programs, July 10, 1969, in *Weekly Compilation of Presidential Documents*, Monday, July 14, 1969.

66. U.S., Department of Health, Education, and Welfare, Social Security Administration, Bureau of Health Insurance, *Health Insurance Benefits Advisory Council Annual Report on Medicare; Covering the Period July 1, 1966 to December 31, 1967* (Washington, D.C.: July 1969), pp. 7–10.

67. "Comparison of Major Features of Peer Review Proposals," Staff Memorandum for HIBAC, HIBAC Agenda Book, July 24–25, 1970, p. 2. Proposed legislation was discussed in HIBAC minutes, XXVII, July 19, 1969, p. 7, and XXIX, November 8, 1969, pp. 13–15. Social Security Amendments proposed in 1969 were not enacted until 1972.

68. *Congressional Record*, July 1, 1970, pp. S10509ff.

69. "Comparison of Major Features of Peer Review Proposals," p. 3.

70. Ibid., pp. 1 and 4.

71. U.S., Congress, Senate, Committee on Finance, Excerpts from Senate Report No. 92-1230, *Report of the Committee on Finance to Accompany H.R. 1, The Social Security Amendments of 1972*, IV, Provisions Relating to Medicare–Medicaid and Maternal and Child Health, 92nd Cong., 2d sess., 1972, p. 256.

72. Ibid., pp. 256-58.

73. Interviews with SSA and BHI officials.

74. Interview with former SSA official involved in legislation. On the Nixon administration and the health care crisis, see chapter 6. For HEW–Finance Committee differences, see "Summary of Differences between Provision Concerning PSROs in Senate Finance Committee Version of H.R. 1 and the Department's Alternative to these Provisions," Finance Committee Staff Paper, October 9, 1972.

75. P.L. 92-603, Section 249 F.

76. Interview with a participant in the legislative process. The distribution of authority also had much to do with concurrent efforts of the secretary and the assistant secretary for health to obtain greater control over the Medicare program. Development of PSRO and utilization review regulations after 1972 reflected conflict between these offices and SSA, but these devleopments are beyond the scope of the study. For policy developments in general, see *Washington Report on Medicine and Health* (Washington, D.C.: McGraw Hill), a weekly newsletter on health policy.

Paying the Hospitals: The Development of Principles of Hospital Reimbursement

When Congress was debating Medicare, much of the nation's hospital care was purchased by insurers, or third-party payers, rather than by individual consumers. Some insurers paid for hospital care as individuals would, that is, according to a hospital bill for services rendered.[1] But by 1965, the largest third-party payer, Blue Cross, generally paid not what a hospital charged for its services, but what it had cost the hospital to provide those services.[2] "Cost reimbursement," as it is called, began on a large scale with the United States Children's Bureau before World War II; spread throughout the country with the Emergency Maternity and Infant Care Program for dependents of servicemen; and was adopted by other federal programs and Blue Cross plans in the 1940s and 1950s. In 1953 the American Hospital Association officially endorsed cost reimbursement in their "Principles of Payment for Hospital Care." By the time Medicare was enacted, hospitals, private insurers, and government officials agreed that hospitals should be paid on the basis of costs.[3] Along with a promise to rely on the expertise and principles of hospitals and private insurers,[4] the law specified that Medicare would pay hospitals the reasonable cost[5] of providing services to beneficiaries.[6]

Agreement to pay costs, however, did not constitute agreement on how to define and measure costs. Specifically, Medicare administrators had to decide how hospitals would compute the share of their total cost attributable to Medicare beneficiaries, and which of the hospitals' costs to include or "allow" as costs of delivering services. There was some controversy on these issues when Congress considered Medicare legislation; drug companies were afraid of limits on payments for trade-name drugs and the insurance industry feared that their beneficiaries would have to cover what Medicare did not.[7] Hospitals and legislators, however, were generally confident that Medicare would improve hospital finances by eliminating the need for charity care. As Wilbur Mills, then chairman of the Ways and Means Committee, explained:

The way it works today, as I understand it, if a hospital succeeds . . . somebody has to pay the costs of operating that hospital during the course of a year. If they don't get it, they go around and ask people to make contributions perhaps, but my thought about it was this: That if you reduced the numbers of those that the hospitals must take care of on a charity basis, as has been done to some extent, even under the present MAA program, if you relieved the hospital of that loss it must charge to the paying patient, that wouldn't result in the transfer of any additional burden to the paying patient. You would take off part of this burden.

In conversation with Social Security Commissioner Robert Ball, Mills observed that the hospitals appeared satisfied to break even. Ball agreed, adding that hospitals favored reasonable costs as an improvement over the present below-cost payment they were receiving for people sixty-five and over. The administration's position, shared by Mills, was that in large part the program would pay for patients who had previously been unable to pay, thereby reducing the need for subsidy from patients under sixty-five and improving the financial position of the hospitals.[8]

When it came time to implement the law, however, hospital confidence waned. The hospitals recognized that the Medicare payments would constitute a major portion of their income and would influence the policies of other third-party payers. Fearing underpayment and seeking financial security for its members, the AHA changed its payment principles and launched a campaign for more liberal definition of "costs" than the law had anticipated.[9]

Medicare's definition of costs had major implications for the program, taxpayers, and consumers. First, meeting the hospitals' demands would make Medicare cost more than predicted. Because Medicare's hospital insurance was financed with an earmarked payroll tax, this excess would require a tax increase. Furthermore, greater hospital revenues could stimulate an upward spiral in Medicare costs in particular and hospital costs in general. If Medicare reimbursement exceeded a hospital's actual expenditures, it would provide the hospital net income to invest in growth and expansion as it saw fit. The capital and operating costs associated with this expansion would then become part of the actual expense third parties would pay in subsequent years.

Whether and on what terms Medicare would finance hospital growth was thus a key element in payment policy. Were SSA pursuing a balancing strategy, officials would have weighed the political advantages of satisfying the hospitals against the disadvantages of higher costs and arrived at a compromise position. Alternatively, had they followed a cost-effectiveness strategy, Medicare officials would have considered the impact of payment on hospital expansion and developed a policy that would inhibit autonomous hospital growth.

In fact, officials in SSA's Bureau of Health Insurance *did* consider the impact of payment policy on Medicare costs, both in the short and long run, and developed payment principles consistent with their view of cost-effectiveness and the public interest. When these proposals failed to satisfy hospital demands, however, SSA's preeminent concern with hospital cooperation, reinforced by the consultation process, led to a compromise that contributed to and legitimized the excessive expenditures BHI had tried to avoid.

Allocating Costs to Medicare

Because Medicare, like Blue Cross, bought only a portion of any hospital's services, it was responsible for only a portion of each hospital's costs. Unlike

Blue Cross, however, the patients Medicare covered were not typical of a hospital's general population. This meant that the way Blue Cross calculated its payment liability was inappropriate for Medicare. Most Blue Cross plans assumed that their subscribers were "average" users of hospital services and, accordingly, paid a hospital its average costs per patient day times the number of days plan subscribers used the hospital. But the elderly, whom Medicare insured, were not average hospital users. They stayed in the hospital longer than other patients and used fewer specialized services per day. As a result the average daily cost of their care was significantly lower than the average for all patients.[10]

The American Hospital Association first brought this fact to congressional attention in 1959, and from that point lower-than-average daily costs were incorporated in Medicare cost estimates.[11] Although Blue Cross expressed some concern about new methods for allocating hospital costs to Medicare,[12] Congress made clear that Medicare should pay its full share of costs and no more by requiring that payment regulations

take into account both direct and indirect costs of providers of services in order that, under the methods of determining costs, the costs with respect to individuals covered by the insurance program established by this title will not be borne by the individuals not so covered, and the costs with respect to individuals not so covered will not be borne by such insurance programs . . .[13]

With this in mind, BHI officials began exploring an alternative to average per diem allocation even before Medicare's enactment. They wanted to find a more accurate measure of beneficiaries' share of costs than the days spent in the hospital. If they could have "counted" the services received and identified exactly the cost of each service, the sum would have been Medicare's payment liability. But services were not so easily measured, nor costs so easily identified. In the absence of other data, BHI officials proposed to use charges for services received as a measure of hospital use. The Ratio of Charges to Costs (RCC)[14] method treats the ratio of charges for beneficiaries' services to charges for all patients as equivalent to beneficiaries' share of the service costs.

Because hospital charges are neither directly nor consistently related to hospital costs, this measure is only approximate. If for example a hospital's charges, relative to its costs, are higher for departments or services that the elderly use heavily than for those they use only slightly, the elderly's share of charges exceeds their actual share of costs. This distortion is reduced, though not eliminated, if the ratio is developed and applied to each hospital department individually. To allocate costs by departmental RCC, a hospital calculates the costs of each department that delivers medical services (revenue-producing departments), for example, radiology, or the operating room; adds to them a share of overhead costs (non-revenue-producing departments); and then multiplies by beneficiaries' share of departmental charges. Compared to average per diem allocation, departmental RCC offered Medicare a more accurate determination of beneficiaries' share of costs, more information on hospital costs in general, and lower program expenditures.[15]

Such advantages to Medicare were disadvantages to the hospitals. Despite their previous acknowledgement that average per diem allocation was inappropriate for the elderly, they found the prospect of less money and new accounting procedures decidedly unappealing. The AHA pressed Medicare to adopt average per diem on the grounds

(1) that the technical difficulties of precise cost finding for the aged were prohibitive, at least for the immediate future; (2) the hidden extra costs of care for the elderly, for which they had never been charged, (were) so great that they might not only fully counterbalance their lesser daily use of ancillaries (nonroutine services) but might, if fully calculated, show that their costs are actually greater than the average.[16]

In preparing policy recommendations for HIBAC, BHI rejected the hospitals' argument. There was no data to support AHA claims of "hidden extra costs," and BHI believed that hospitals could adopt "more modern procedures" of accounting.[17]

The fact that average cost per day has been used for a number of years and hospitals are familiar with it, should not be a barrier against the use of any other relatively simple procedure which results in a more correct cost determination of the actual services received. Hospitals in a relatively short period of time can also become familiar with other relatively simple procedures. The important fact is that whatever procedure is used it should serve to insure full value for the funds paid out for services.[18]

BHI officials therefore recommended to HIBAC that Medicare adopt departmental RCC.[19] To give hospitals time to adjust to this new[20] and relatively sophisticated accounting method, they proposed to allow hospitals the simpler alternative of applying RCC to total rather than departmental costs (the gross RCC method) for one or two years, with the understanding that Medicare would then require departmental cost calculations. Hospitals that could not manage gross RCC at the start of the program could use other methods for short periods. Intermediaries, state agencies, and "other appropriate sources" would provide consultative services "to enable providers to tool up within a reasonable period" to use departmental RCC.[21] The objective, according to BHI Director Arthur Hess, was to come as close as possible to actual cost by using the best method possible for a particular institution at a particular time, thereby generally improving hospital accounting and cost determination.[22]

As they consulted with HIBAC and the industry, however, BHI was willing to compromise this objective. Although HIBAC agreed with BHI that RCC was the most accurate apportionment formula and the one most consistent with congressional intent, they were concerned about hospitals' difficulties in meeting its recordkeeping requirements. In their deliberations, they sought to balance accuracy with simplicity, while avoiding what the HIBAC minutes describe as potential "inequities" in hospital payment. One "inequity" that concerned Council members was paying hospitals *less* than their actual costs. To avoid it, the Council rejected apportionment methods that relied on averages and did not compute each hospital's costs individually. But the Council was prepared to pay hospitals *more* than their actual costs to avoid the "inequity" of paying some hospitals less than others.[23] A senior SSA official explained how a general requirement for sophisticated accounting, with allowances for particular hospital problems, could create a policy problem: "If you give a financial break to a hospital because it doesn't keep good books, you penalize the good guy."[24] To prevent this "inequity" the Council decided

to offer hospitals an option between a method relatively easy for all hospitals to implement and a method that would more accurately reflect the cost of services provided to medicare patients.[25]

This decision gave hospitals an opportunity to choose the method that offered greater reimbursement, regardless of their ability to determine Medicare's actual costs.

The options HIBAC recommended and BHI adopted were (1) departmental RCC and (2) a combination method using average per diem for room and board and gross RCC for nonroutine or ancillary services. Regulations included no time limits on availability of options and no requirement for departmental RCC at some future date.[26]

A BHI official responsible for payment regulations explained why the agency did not require departmental RCC. BHI did not agree with the industry that hospitals could not undertake departmental RCC. On the contrary, this official recalled, in field investigations "we found the technicians could do it, but their spokesmen didn't know it." Nevertheless, BHI, with HIBAC encouragement, was anxious to mitigate the fears these spokesmen expressed. By allowing hospitals accounting options, administrators believed they could boost hospital "morale"—and achieve industry acceptance of accurate accounting principles. Time limits were considered inappropriate to this effort. Besides, this official added, the 1965–1966 regulations were to be a starting point, subject to review and revision in the future.[27]

Capital Reimbursement

As reimbursement negotiations continued, however, BHI departed further from requirements for precise and accurate allocation. Somers and Somers, who observed early Medicare policymaking at first hand, explained that despite the appearance of "discrete and relatively independent" regulations, "in reimbursement bargaining they are, in effect, a package."[28] No part of this package received greater attention than reimbursement for hospitals' capital costs.

Most observers of the long reimbursement negotiations agree that the hospitals' drive to increase funds for capital formation colored and complicated every major dispute on payment. It intruded upon consideration of items, where it seemed relevant and where it did not, and proved to be the hospitals' most effective weapon in obtaining various liberalizations.[29]

Before Medicare, hospitals obtained about one-third of the capital they used for maintenance and growth from patient revenues. The rest came from grants from all levels of government, donations, and borrowing.[30] If the hospitals could obtain capital payments in Medicare reimbursement, they could greatly enhance their fiscal stability and freedom to spend. Given Medicare's decision to certify most of the nation's hospitals for participation, capital payments through reimbursement would provide almost all hospitals with the wherewithal for maintenance and expansion. In designing capital reimbursement, Medicare administrators therefore had to decide to what extent their program would finance the nation's hospital system.

Hospitals first raised the capital question with respect to the timing of Medicare payments. They expressed concern about having adequate funds or "working capital" to cover expenses they incurred before they got paid. When BHI officials responded with an offer to pay hospitals before instead of after they delivered services,[31] it became apparent that timing was only a small part of the hospitals' concern. Their primary objective was to obtain additional revenue in two areas: (1) the definition of Medicare payments for depreciation on buildings and equipment; and (2) the inclusion of a return on equity as an allowable cost.

Depreciation is an accounting device to reflect an asset's decline in value over the years it is used. Firms attribute a portion of their income to asset depreciation to reflect their net worth more accurately. This accounting practice involves no cash outlay; depreciation allowances are "simply subtractions from overstated asset figures. . . ."[32] But tax deductions for depreciation or depreciation payments provide income that allows recovery of the firm's initial investment over time. The income recovered is not obligated in any way and is available to use as the firm sees fit.

These characteristics of depreciation present some problems when applied to nonprofit hospitals. First of all, depreciation payments justified as recovery of investment are appropriate only if the payments go to the original investor. This would not apply to the significant portion of nonprofit hospital investment financed through public and private grants.[33] Second, even if depreciation is alternatively justified as payment for using up assets that belong to the hospital, its reimbursement differs from other cost reimbursement because no expenditure has been made. Hence, what the hospital will do with the funds is an open question.

Even before Medicare, hospitals and third parties had answered this question by deciding that since depreciation made funds available for capital replacement, that was what it ought to do.[34] In essence, the consequences of depreciation reimbursement had become its justification.

With Medicare, the hospitals took their rationale one step further.[35] Before 1965, almost all third parties who paid depreciation did so according to traditional business accounting procedures, that is, based on the original or historical costs of assets. But when Medicare began, the hospitals took a new tack. They now argued that if depreciation was supposed to provide capital for replacement and expansion, it should be more liberally defined. Accordingly, one month after Medicare was enacted, the AHA changed its Principles for Payment to endorse depreciation based on current or replacement costs rather than original costs of assets.[36]

HIBAC deliberations generated a second way to provide capital through Medicare reimbursement. Starting with the notion that it might be "inequitable" to pay interest on borrowed capital, as the law specified, without paying "imputed interest" on contributed capital, the Council directed BHI to consider paying the hospitals "interest" or a return on their assets.[37] This can be equated with profit,[38] but because the law allowed reimbursement only for costs, attention turned to its justification as a "cost of capital," that is, the interest those funds could have earned if invested elsewhere. This interest could be construed as what an enterprise might have to pay to attract capital investment or to borrow money. But since a hospital that received capital through public grants or private donations in fact incurred no such cost, to reimburse for it would provide hospitals with an unobligated accretion to income, as depreciation would.

Reinforcing these payment proposals was a consensus in the industry and in the health field that hospitals faced enormous needs for capital that Medicare could help meet. Early in their deliberations, HIBAC's chairman, Kermit Gordon, summed up the sense of the Council that "the principles governing cost reimbursement under the hospital insurance program should treat the future capital needs of health facilities as generously as possible."[39] Similarly, a Public Health Service task force argued that Medicare was supported by tax money, constituted community resources for health care, and should contribute generously to the support of institutions used by its beneficiaries.[40] A close observer of the policy process recalled that most of the health care experts, as well as industry, believed that Medicare should give hospitals money so that they could improve care.[41]

This belief assumes that what is good for each hospital is good for the public. But deciding what is good for the public requires an assessment of the benefits of hospital expansion in relation to its costs. If cost reimbursement provides hospitals with capital to expand services, no one makes such an assessment. The hospital can expand as it sees fit, free from all cost constraints. Patients are not concerned about costs their insurer pays; they and their physicians seek the most sophisticated care available.[42] Even if a hospital has too few patients to use its services to capacity, it obtains revenue to support them by allocating service costs to the patients it does have, and to the third parties that insure them.[43] There is no place in this payment system to evaluate whether the services hospitals provide and insurance supports are worth what they cost.

BHI Opposition

BHI officials recognized this problem in developing positions on reimbursement for capital expenditures. They found the proposals made by HIBAC and the hospitals contrary to the public interest in influence and control over hospital expenditures and in excess of Medicare's cost estimates. They therefore proposed to define Medicare's capital payments far more narrowly than the hospitals advocated.

Because the committee reports mentioned depreciation as a reasonable cost, BHI did not question its inclusion in reimbursement.[44] But they did question how it should be defined and calculated. First of all, they rejected the AHA's demand for current-cost depreciation. That method, they argued, was used in only two or three areas of the country, was contrary to most business and accounting practices, and would raise Medicare's depreciation costs from 6 percent of total reimbursement to 9 percent. Furthermore,

"Although capital is still needed for more acute bed facilities in some areas, so much bed expansion had been financed that overbuilding is now identified as a dangerous threat to the quality of care." This point raises the issue of how can the Government finance replacement of needed facilities without paying for unnecessary replacement or expansion? The staff (BHI) is very concerned about the effect of setting a national policy which would encourage the replacement or construction of hospitals without a regard to whether they were needed.[45]

On these grounds, they proposed to use historical cost depreciation, calculated uniformly over the life of an asset, that is, by the straight-line method.[46]

Secondly, based on the committee reports, BHI found it in their discretion to question whether Medicare should pay depreciation on federally financed, or Hill-Burton, hospital assets.[47] On the grounds that such payments would mean the federal government had paid twice for the same asset, once through Hill-Burton and again through depreciation, BHI concluded that "over the long run, the program should not provide an allowance for depreciation of Hill-Burton assets."[48]

This viewpoint is supported by a recent Bureau of Budget Directive prohibiting allowances for depreciation under certain contracts for the cost of any portion of an asset that was financed or donated by the Federal Government.[49]

Apparently because Blue Cross reimbursement for depreciation had included Hill-Burton assets, however, BHI proposed a "grandfather clause," permitting depreciation payments on Hill-Burton assets acquired before July 1, 1966, Medicare's starting date.

Since all hospitals would be on notice that depreciation would not be allowed with respect to the Hill-Burton portion of assets acquired on or after 7/1/66, it would not be inequitable in view of this period of reasonable notice to disallow depreciation on such assets.[50]

When it came to imputed interest or "cost of capital," BHI was more emphatic that capital payments through reimbursement were neither in keeping with the law nor efficient policy for hospital development. They explored "imputed interest" at the Council's direction and estimated its costs as an additional $100 million, or 3 to 4 percent in the program's first year. In arguing against it, they first explained that there was no "cost of capital" for non-profit hospitals:

A businessman who invests in a hospital provides risk capital invested as a business venture. The interest he could have received is, from an economic standpoint, a cost the businessman incurs for using his own money to finance capital goods. While the language of the law precludes payments under the program to include an allowance for profit, it might be reasonable to reimburse the entrepreneur for the economic cost of lost interest.

It would appear that imputed interest does not represent an item of economic cost for the nonprofit provider. The funds that nonprofit providers receive from the community are contributed for the sole purpose of making health services available to the community; the community does not view that hospital as one of a number of alternative possible money-making ventures. Since the funds so collected are generally not intended for, and cannot be put to, an alternative use which will earn a financial return, there is no basis for recognizing economic cost from loss of interest.[51]

Second, they reiterated their arguments that providing capital through Medicare reimbursement was "a wasteful and inefficient form of subsidy for the construction and improvement of health care facilities": (1) Payments would be related to the elderly proportion of the hospital's population rather than its need for capital. (2) By enabling the hospital to accumulate a large capital reserve, such reimbursement

might over the long run make hospitals independent of community interest. Selective perpetuation may be desired and even required, but blanket perpetuation which produce [sic] unnecessary facilities should not be encouraged.[52]

(3) This approach would undermine federal and local hospital planning efforts to allocate funds for changing community needs. And (4)

Indiscriminate funancing of health care facilities will add to the cost of care in three ways: (1) The spending of the money necessary to create unneeded facilities; (2) The expense of operating under conditions of below-optimum usage; and (3) The unneeded or unduly prolonged hospital care which will result from the tendency to relax admission and discharge standards to maximize the hospitals' income in order to meet expenses. More important than economic considerations is the fact that unnecessary hospital or medical care may be a danger to the patient.[53]

For all these reasons, BHI argued that federal funds for construction and replacement of hospitals should not be provided through Medicare. Instead they should be channelled through a program, like Hill-Burton, that would "gear subsidies to need."[54]

HIBAC agreed not to recommend current-cost depreciation, but advocated more liberal calculations than BHI had proposed, and, along with the hospitals, continued to press BHI to consider imputed interest.[55] The agency remained opposed to imputed interest and made a case to the Council against it. First, they presented substantial data on the capital that hospitals could accumulate if they funded their depreciation payments, that is, placed them in a separate account restricted to use for capital purposes.[56] Although officials did not expect the hospitals to do this, they believed that the possibility was a good argument against additional reimbursement.[57] BHI estimated that if hospitals funded 95 percent of their depreciation payments over the next twenty-five years, reserves would then equal almost half the value of total assets. Second, officials told HIBAC, imputed interest calculations would impose on Medicare the tremendous problems of public utility regulation, such as establishing an asset base, and again raise the question of how to treat government-financed capital. Citing a New York regulatory commission finding "that a telephone company which is primarily financed with low-cost federal money should not be permitted to profit on such funds at the expense of its subscribers," BHI suggested that the ruling would similarly apply to the "no-cost Federal money" that hospitals used.[58]

To strengthen their case against capital financing through Medicare reimbursement, BHI officials sought support elsewhere in HEW.[59] Dr. William Stewart, Surgeon General and head of HEW's "health" activities, made a presentation to HIBAC against current-cost depreciation.[60] After giving evidence on the unequal distribution of health facilities around the country, Dr. Stewart emphasized that capital through reimbursement would do little to rectify this situation. Capital reimbursement based on plant value would give the most capital to the hospitals that already had the newest and best plant, and to the states with most facilities.

This is both a national and a community problem. Public effort is increasingly directed to area-wide planning for the development of health services and facilities. Needs change, populations move. But a hospital board with money in its pocket can be expected to be more concerned with its institutional future than with the broad needs of the community. Unless those charged with an overview of community health needs have some financial leverage to help develop facilities geared to needs, the hospital rich will get richer and the poor will get poorer.[61]

Furthermore, Dr. Stewart observed, they would do so at the expense of the nation's poor people.

Under hospital insurance, be it Social Security, Blue Cross, or any other—rich and poor pay equally for presumably equal benefits. But when capital depreciation factors are added to the insurance cost, rich and poor are paying equal shares of very expensive capital expenditures. The regressiveness of this taxing becomes more important as the proportion of the total capital so financed increases.[62]

Negotiating a Compromise

These arguments did not convince hospitals, HIBAC, or even senior Medicare officials that Medicare should not provide capital for hospitals. "Imputed interest just cost too much," explained a senior SSA official. Had a return on equity not required a tax increase, observers and participants recall, Medicare would probably have paid it.[63] A council member who opposed capital reimbursement characterized HIBAC's debate by recounting an exchange with a member who favored it: "He told me," said the first, "that I'd end up with a beautiful trust fund and no hospitals. And I told him he'd have beautiful hospitals and no money to buy services from them."[64] Although capital advocates were in the majority on the council, the prospect of program costs in the first year amounting to 6 to 8 percent or $150–200 million more than estimated, and therefore a tax increase before the program even started, constrained their generosity.[65] Based on these costs, Commissioner Ball pressed the council not to deal with Medicare as the major source of hospital capital,[66] and the council agreed to compromise. They decided to hold back a recommendation for imputed interest for one year, at which time the issue would be reconsidered in light of the hospitals' financial position.[67] In a letter to the secretary, the council expressed their belief that

The Medicare program, insofar as the law allows, should be administered in such fashion as to help on a pro rata basis to strengthen the financial position of these institutions, in order to improve their ability to maintain, renovate, and replace their capital facilities. . . .

The Council must record for you its grave concern with regard to the financing needs of our nation's health care·system. It is obvious that the cost of patient care cannot currently include a cost factor to provide for unknown needs, but it is also obvious that current costs cannot and should not ignore the financing that is necessary to avoid deterioration in the present level of patient care.[68]

In closing, the letter made clear that other government action to support health care facilities would affect its considerations, noting finally that "the important point is that our institutional health care system not deteriorate and that its capital needs be recognized and met."[69]

Just as the council accepted SSA's argument on costs, SSA accepted the council's and the industry's commitment to additional capital. Unable to sell their position, a BHI official explained, or to promote an alternative strategy in HEW for federal financing for hospitals,[70] BHI found ways to provide capital through reimbursement within the constraints of program financing. Although they held the line on imputed interest, BHI adjusted their depreciation policy to provide the hospitals with additional revenue. The estimated cost of these changes for Medicare's first year was approximately $120 million more than predicted, but leeway in program cost projections made these funds available without a tax increase.[71] Justifications for policies varied, but SSA increasingly adopted the rationales for capital reimbursement that BHI had originally rejected.

To provide hospitals with "working capital," Medicare would pay all hospitals before rather than after they delivered services.[72] To help hospitals acquire capital to pay off mortgages or to accumulate reserves for replacement, Medicare would pay depreciation on an accelerated rather than a straight-line basis.[73] This would mean bigger payments in earlier years, on which the hospital could accumulate interest if it chose.[74] To accommodate hospitals that lacked original cost records without "penalizing" hospitals that *had* cost records, Medicare would allow all hospitals to estimate their depreciation costs for assets acquired before 1966 at 5 percent of 1965 operating costs. This option would disappear by reducing that percentage 0.5 percent per year.[75] Finally, "to replace a used up asset" regardless of its financing and "to provide funds which make it possible to keep the asset or its future equivalent permanently,"[76] Medicare would pay depreciation on all Hill-Burton financed assets, before and after 1966.[77]

In agreeing to provide these capital payments to hospitals, Medicare had one route left that might prevent the wasteful expenditures they predicted hospitals would make. Medicare officials had to decide whether to require that depreciation be funded, making reserves available for capital replacement when it became necessary, and whether to regulate expenditures from the funds, for example, by tying expenditures to community planning. In discussing hospitals' need for capital, HIBAC members expressed concern about potential waste and requested that SSA investigate its legal authority to make such requirements.[78] On the advice of legal counsel, the agency concluded that it lacked this authority.[79]

Interviews suggest that this interpretation of the law reflected other administrative judgments, which were somewhat contradictory. First of all, despite the above rationale for depreciation on Hill-Burton assets, officials continued to question the wisdom of a funding requirement that would "assure each hospital the ability to operate in perpetuity."[80] But they might have followed the "logic" of capital provisions by requiring funding had it not been for other considerations. In 1965, most hospitals did not follow the recommendation of the AHA and hospital financing experts that they fund depreciation. Instead, they spent depreciation reimbursement as it came along. BHI chose not to interfere with existing practices. "Had we interfered with hospital flexibility by tying up depreciation money," said a BHI official, "we'd have brought down an avalanche on our entire payment system."[81] A funding requirement with a planning requirement would have been an even greater limitation on that flexibility.[82] Therefore, on the grounds that depreciation payments were part of reasonable costs,[83] SSA decided they had no authority to regulate their use. Despite the above reservations, however, they were willing to encourage funding by agreeing not to deduct interest earned on depreciation funds from reimbursable costs.[84] In sum, SSA's inconsistent policies were consistent in making payments to the hospitals with no strings attached.

With HIBAC agreement on allocation and capital, and the payment concessions they had made in these and other areas, SSA thought they had a reimbursement policy that the hospitals would accept. But in mid-April 1965, just before SSA was ready to make regulations public, the AHA balked. According to an SSA official, an AHA representative reported: "I can't sell them what we've agreed to."[85] A contemporary account of the hospitals' attitude refers to a "stormy meeting" at AHA headquarters in Chicago in mid-April:

With Arthur E. Hess, Director of SSA's Bureau, Health Insurance, present, state association leaders—particularly those from California—obtained assurance that AHA would made a last ditch fight with government about the reimbursement proposals.

Following that meeting, Avery M. Millard, executive director of the California Hospital Association, commented, "We are very glad that the AHA is taking the initiative at this point, because our feeling was one of strong disappointment as to how our hospitals would fare. It was going to be necessary to do something within the democratic process to provide some relief."

Reportedly, the Chicago meeting was followed by immediate overtures by a number of state delegations with their Congressmen, and this in turn was reported as materially influencing the concessions granted in the week following the conference.[86]

To get those concessions, the hospitals had to go over SSA's head to HEW undersecretary Wilbur Cohen and Secretary John Gardner. The hospitals demanded average per diem allocation and a specific payment for capital. SSA and their superiors in HEW would not give in to either of these demands in full.

Instead they lumped the two together as the justification for a "plus factor" in reimbursement, that is, the addition to each hospital's Medicare reimbursement of 2 percent of its identified allowable cost.[87] BHI proposed to justify the plus factor as a payment for capital, or "to maintain an institution's service rendering capability in the face of technological advance."[88] This was the way the hospitals understood the payment, referring to it as a "capital improvement payment."[89] Commissioner Ball emphasized the capital factor in explaining the payment to HIBAC, but added other elements as well:

After long and careful deliberation, during which the Council's conclusion that the case for payment for the use of equity capital had considerable merit as well as the representations of the AHA were considered, a decision was made to allow, as an element of reasonable cost for both proprietary and non-proprietary providers, a payment equal to 2 percent of the cost otherwise allowed (with the exception of interest expense), subject to the limitation that this allowance not exceed a reasonable long-term interest rate on the provider's equity capital. This allowance is partly in lieu of a direct interest return on the equity capital of providers and partly in recognition of the lack of precision in cost finding in the early stages of program operation, as well as being in lieu of other elements of cost not specifically recognized.[90]

These "other elements" were the "hidden extra costs" that the hospitals attributed to routine services for the elderly, and for which they had sought average per diem allocation.[91]

Thus, Medicare policy had come full circle. From a position emphasizing precise cost measurement and limited capital payments, they had shifted to acceptance of the hospitals' claims, disputing only how much to pay for them. As Commissioner Ball explained to HIBAC, the plus factor had made reimbursement more responsive to hospitals' needs and would cost the program only 2 percent rather than the 10 percent associated with average per diem and a return on equity.[92]

It is clear from this account that Medicare policy was not made without consideration of its impact on hospital growth and development. The negative consequences of liberal reimbursement were enumerated, considered, and rejected as the primary determinant of policy. Why? Partly because senior SSA and HEW officials accepted the consensus in the health field that hospital "improvement" was a good thing, to which the payment concession made only a small contribution. But even they would have been less generous if the hospitals had not pressed them. What made these officials and even BHI opponents of capital reimbursement respond to that pressure was their commitment to a "proper takeoff" for Medicare. Some observers have said that Medicare officials feared a hospital boycott if they did not give in. The officials themselves explain their position differently. Their feeling, according to a senior SSA official, was that the hospitals would have to go along with whatever rules the department promulgated. "But there's a real difference in launching a program with the help of the hospitals as opposed to against them. To an administrator, that difference makes all the difference in the world." A BHI official expressed a similar point of view: The hospitals were not "our adversaries; we were all in the same lifeboat together."[93]

If the hospitals perceived SSA policy as "fair, not generous but fair,"[94] administrators believed they would cooperate in implementing the law, for example, by integrating their hospitals, performing paperwork, and giving Medicare favorable publicity. A BHI official explained, "We didn't want headlines that SSA was going to drive the hospitals out of business."[95] With the final concessions in reimbursement, SSA turned the AHA and its members from potential antagonists into allies in Medicare implementation. Thus when Ball announced the reimbursement principles, complimenting the AHA on its "vigorous presentation of the hospital case," the AHA executive vice-president, Dr. Edwin Crosby, responded with praise for the "understanding, cooperation and patience of the commissioner and his staff."[96] Shortly thereafter, the AHA House of Delegates passed a special resolution urging "all hospitals to participate in the implementation of Public Law 89–97 (Social Security Amendments of 1965)."[97]

Now SSA had the cooperation of the hospitals, but the concessions they had made to win it aroused the ire of a congressional committee that had to pay for them. The Senate Finance Committee charged that HEW had exceeded its authority by promising to pay the hospitals $750 million over the next ten years for purposes Congress had neither considered nor approved.[98] Some senators felt that HEW had negotiated a deal with the hospitals without adequately consulting them.[99] Committee staff members had had difficulty obtaining minutes of the HIBAC meetings, for example.[100] Senator Clinton Anderson (D-New Mexico) was most outspoken in disapproving HEW's actions, and, as a sponsor of Medicare bills throughthe 1960's, expressed a sense of betrayal at the reimbursement principles:

We had a good deal of discussion about this bill and many people talked about its unsoundness before it was even adopted, the dangers inherent in it, the fact that costs would get too high. And Bob Myers made estimates as to how the thing would work out.

Over a long period of years we have trusted the estimates and relied on them tremendously, and I did then and do now.

But after he got through with his estimates, new things were introduced. And now how many things are going to be added?

Will there be 10 percent added finally? You said it is an issue you are going to study. Why don't you wait for 1 year and find out what the real facts are, which you don't have now any more than you had before.

Why don't you wait to settle this question until there is a chance to settle it?[101]

The committee and its staff challenged the reimbursement principles on much the same grounds that BHI had originally advocated more restricted reimbursement—that unregulated payments to the hospitals for expenses they had not actually incurred would produce wasteful, expensive, and inefficient hospital growth. Thus the staff proposed that depreciation not be paid on publicly financed assets or, if paid, that regulations require that it be funded; and that the 2 percent "bonus" be eliminated from reimbursement.[102]

The senators were not in agreement on these issues. Senator Anderson strongly opposed the "sweeteners" he felt SSA had added to anticipated reimbursement,[103] while Senator Paul Douglas (D-Illinois) advocated Medicare reimbursement for hospital growth and development.[104] But the senators shared a concern about paying depreciation and a plus factor without constraints on hospitals' use of the funds.[105]

In general, Cohen and Ball defended their reimbursement principles as legitimate reflections of hospital costs.[106] Although it conflicted with their own justification of depreciation on Hill-Burton assets, they agreed emphatically with the senators' concerns about potentially uncontrolled hospital expansion. They proposed, however, that such controls be developed in other legislation, arguing that there was no authority in the Medicare law to control hospitals' expenditures.[107] Senator Anderson disagreed with their interpretation:

I would say when there is no prohibition on putting controls on these things, you ought to try to put it on, and let somebody take it into court and see if they can take it off. I think they would have a hard time doing it. But at least you would have tried to do something that is in accordance with ordinary, reasonable, precautions; namely if they are going to get money to replace buildings it ought to be for approved construction or equipment. Otherwise you are going to have a cancer machine in every hospital, regardless of need.[108]

Senator Anderson preferred that they wait to put the money into hospitals until it was needed. He said, "You are going to put the money in now and settle the question in advance. That is what most of us are worried about."[109]

Here and elsewhere Cohen offered another argument with which Medicare officials generally defended their reimbursement decisions: that they had taken a *conservative* position on payment and made a good bargain on the government's behalf.[110]

Mr. Cohen: . . . I think you also have to keep in mind that the hospitals did come in and make representation to Mr. Ball and the Secretary for proposals which were very substantially beyond what we are now talking about in the guidelines that we issued. . . .
Mr. Ball: They had the idea that two percent would be desirable, that it would be desirable to also have depreciation on a replacement basis, that it would be desirable to have the average per diem. And the only point in dispute that we later agreed with them on—in major cost matters—and then on a different rationale than theirs (i.e. not imputed interest) was the two percent. . . .
Mr. Cohen: I thought, Senator, having sat in many conference committees that one side asked for 19 and we settled for 2, was a very, very reasonable conservative solution.[111]

Senator Anderson did not share their persepctive; he insisted, "No great problem is settled until it is settled right. If they asked for something wrong, 2 percent is as bad as 19 percent. I know you believe in the compromise. But sometimes we don't."[112] Senator Douglas (D-Illinois) had a different point of view. He replied to Senator Anderson's suggestion that SSA wait to evaluate hospital need before offering concessions:

> If we are getting into practical considerations, let me say you have to give the hospitals a little grease to operate when they make the transition.
> The wheels won't turn unless the axle has a little grease. And if there is grease in this—and I think in the long run there is not grease—if there should be grease, I would not object to a little grease the first year. Grease has been known to perform very useful functions in other branches of the Government, I don't know why it cannot perform a useful function in Medicare. . . .[113]

"Practical considerations" more than resolution of the issues kept SSA's payment agreement intact. The senators were keenly aware,[114] and Ball and Cohen made certain to remind them, that

> it is now 36 days away from the date that Medicare must start, and most of the hospitals that want to make agreements with us have not signed written agreements pending our formal promulgation of these principles as regulations.
> I would merely like to say to the Senator (Long), since our procedures are to issue them as proposed regulations, giving people 30 days' notice to comment, it was our proposal now to go ahead and issue the proposed regulations in the Federal Register, subject to the 30 days for comment, so that we might be able, within those 30 days, still to get the hospitals to sign an agreement and meet the July 1 deadline. And I thought I had better say that to the Senator before he left the hearing room because I think unless we give the other people throughout the country the opportunity to make their comments and criticisms in the 30 day period, we cannot sign up the hospitals in order to go into effect on July 1.[115]

According to a legislative participant, time decided the matter.[116] Regardless of reservations, there was simply not enough time to change the program before it was scheduled to begin. In fact, the only major change the committee did impose,[117] using legislation to do it, required Medicare to liberalize its reimbursement for proprietary institutions.[118] Thus, in their desire to get Medicare smoothly underway and their willingness to pay the hospitals for cooperation, at least in one area, the Senate Finance Committee and the Congress essentially reinforced SSA's strategy on reimbursement.

Even if SSA had not compromised with the hospitals, Medicare would probably have increased hospital net income and expenditures, simply by paying for care that the elderly had not previously paid for or even received. This was a product of the Medicare legislation, not administrative discretion. But where they had discretion, administrators consciously subordinated fiscal control to hospital cooperation, thereby fueling the inflation they had tried to avoid.

Although at least some officials believed that these initial policies could be changed once the program was underway, the following chapters will reveal how SSA's continuing concern with political balance in fact led to their entrenchment.

Notes

1. When the for-profit insurers (in contrast to the nonprofit Blue Cross) pay hospitals directly, they pay on the basis of charges.

2. In the mid-sixties, two-thirds of the Blue Cross plans used cost-related reimbursement formulas. Herman M. Somers and Anne R. Somers, *Medicare and the Hospitals* (Washington, D.C.: The Brookings Institution, 1967), p. 156.

3. This history of cost reimbursement comes from Somers and Somers, *Medicare and the Hospitals*, pp. 154–58 and Irwin Wolkstein, "The Legislative History of Hospital Cost Reimbursement," in U.S., Department of Health, Education, and Welfare, Social Security Administration, Office of Research and Statistics, *Reimbursement Incentives for Hospital and Medical Care: Objectives and Alternatives*, Research Report no. 26 (1968), pp. 1–15 (hereafter cited as Legislative History).

4. Although the AHA accepted legislative provisions on cost reimbursement as adequate assurance that their principles would be observed, AMA criticism led to specification in the 1962 legislative proposal and the final law that Medicare would follow "the principles generally applied by national organizations (that have developed such principles) in computing the amount of payment." Wolkstein, "Legislative History," pp. 8–9. For HEW's explanation of its intentions, see U.S., Congress, House, Committee on Ways and Means, *Medical Care for the Aged: Executive Hearings before the Committee on Ways and Means on H.R. 1 and other Proposals for Medical Care for the Aged*, 89th Cong., 1st sess., 1965, pp. 140, 142, 783–85.

5. The AHA would have preferred "full" to "reasonable costs," but they were not disturbed by the difference. See Committee on Ways and Means, *Medical Care for the Aged*, 1965, pp. 228 and 293. To paraphrase a former AHA official, "They accused us of seeking unreasonable costs. We couldn't have that." The implications of "reasonable" will be discussed in chapter 6.

6. 42 U.S.C. sec. 1395x(v)(1) and Excerpts from Report on Committee on Finance, U.S. Senate, to Accompany H.R. 6675, 1965, pp. 35–37, and Excerpts from Report of the Committee on Ways and Means on H.R. 6675, pp. 31–33, both in New Members Background Book, Part I, for HIBAC, 1968. The law and the committee reports elaborated extensively on the variety of ways in which costs could be calculated.

7. Wolkstein, "Legislative History," p. 9. Commercial insurance companies, in contrast to Blue Cross, frequently insured patients on an indemnity basis, that is, paid a portion of hospital charges. Thus they were quite concerned that any

inadequacies that hospitals found in Medicare reimbursement would be dealt with by increasing charges to paying patients, thereby decreasing the value of their insurance. (Committee on Ways and Means, *Medical Care for the Aged*, 1965, pp. 393 ff.) On the one hand, this concern was directed toward Medicare's approach to allowable costs—that is, would such things as depreciation, obsolescence, charity care, research, and teaching be included in "reasonable costs?" On the other hand, they were concerned about computing the program's share of total costs on any basis other than average per diem for the entire patient population. Blue Cross expressed the latter concern in testimony before the Senate Finance Committee. (U.S., Congress, Senate, Committee on Finance, *Social Security, Hearings on H.R. 6675*, 89th Cong., 1st sess. 1965, pp. 342-43). While they supported cost reimbursement, like the commercial insurance companies, they did not wish the share of hospital costs for which their beneficiaries were held responsible to increase.

8. Committee on Ways and Means, *Medical Care for the Aged*, 1965, pp. 149 and 727.

9. For a discussion of AHA's position and the reimbursement principles, see Somers and Somers, *Medicare and the Hospitals*, chapter 8.

10. Ibid., pp. 166-67.

11. Wolkstein, "Legislative History," pp. 6-7.

12. Committee on Finance, *Hearings on H.R. 6675*, 1965, pp. 342-43. See note 7 above.

13. 42 U.S.C. sec. 1395x(v).

14. This method is actually the Ratio of Charges to Charges Applied to Costs (RCCAC) but at the time was generally referred to as RCC.

15. See discussion in Somers and Somers, *Medicare and the Hospitals*, pp. 168-69. Preliminary results of an AHA-SSA study comparing RCC with average per diem allocation showed a difference of 13 percent. (HIBAC minutes, II, November 21, 1965, p. 12.) Generally the difference was considered to be from 8 to 10 percent. Somers and Somers, p. 167.

16. Ibid.

17. "Average Cost Per Day Formula", p. 13, in HIBAC Agenda Book, December 17-19, 1965.

18. Ibid.

19. Ibid., p. 3.

20. Ibid., p. 3. HIBAC was informed that variations of RCC were understood to be in operation in South Carolina, Massachusetts, and Connecticut and being contemplated for use in Maryland.

21. Ibid.

22. HIBAC Minutes, II, November 21, 1965, p. 13.

23. HIBAC Minutes, IV:1, January 7, 1966, pp. 7-10.

24. Interview.

25. HIBAC Minutes, IV:1, January 7, 1966, p. 10.

26. "Principles of Reimbursement for Provider Costs," Principle 2-2, 20 C.F.R. 405.452. After the first reporting period, a hospital needed its intermediary's permission to switch from one option to the other. The regulations also included temporary options. For eighteen months hospitals using the combination method could estimate rather than compute the distribution of costs between routine and ancillary services, and for one reporting period, providers unable to use any other method could use gross RCC or another "reasonable" method.

27. Interview.

28. Somers and Somers, *Medicare and the Hospitals*, p. 161.

29. Ibid., p. 177.

30. For an analysis of hospitals' capital financing, see Paul B. Ginsburg, "Resource Allocation in the Hospital Industry," *Social Security Bulletin* 35 (October 1972): 20-30.

31. Interviews with BHI officials. BHI officials believed that the interest Medicare would lose in this transaction would be small and less costly than the interest Medicare would have to pay if hospitals borrowed money to cover operating expenses. Furthermore, it would provide for smooth program operation if hospital use significantly increased at the start of the program.

32. See Paul A. Samuelson, *Economics: An Introductory Analysis*, 6th ed. (New York: McGraw Hill, 1964), p. 105.

33. In 1966, private grants accounted for 30.2 percent of voluntary hospitals' capital funds, and government grants, 10.1 percent. See Ginsburg, "Resource Allocations," pp. 22-23.

34. In a letter to the Ways and Means Committee in 1967, H. Sibley, executive director of the Hospital Planning Council for Metropolitan Chicago, offered an explanation of depreciation as a reimbursable cost. He argued that the Medicare regulations follow IRS rules that are based on the premise that investors have the right to recover their original monetary investment over a reasonable period of time. But with hospital reimbursement, there is no intention of permitting hospitals to pay off those who originally made contributions to finance buildings. People knowledgeable of hospital financing, he noted, hold that the depreciation allowance in hospital reimbursement is instead intended to permit the hospital to accumulate reserves for capital cost of modernization, renovation and replacement. U.S. Congress, House, Committee on Ways and Means, *President's Proposals for Revision of the Social Security System: Hearings on H.R. 5710*, 90th Cong., 1st sess., 1967, p. 2277. Sibley was making an argument for current cost depreciation. On third-party depreciation payments, see also Lawrence E. Martin, "Capital Needs for the Facilities of the Voluntary Hospital System," a position paper for the Secretary's Advisory Committee on Hospital Effectiveness, pp. 1-2 (Typewritten).

35. See Somers and Somers, *Medicare and the Hospitals*, p. 172.

36. Ibid., pp. 171-72.

37. HIBAC minutes, II, November 21, 1965, p. 15. A former HIBAC member explained: If the policy were to pay only actual interest and there were two hospitals, one with a large debt and one with substantial equity, they would receive very different payments.

38. In a "Background Statement on Imputed Interest," BHI distinguished between the economic interpretation of profit as compensation for risk (therefore excluding imputed interest) and the accounting definition as "the difference between revenues and the actual costs and expense of obtaining the revenue." HIBAC Agenda Book, December 17-19, 1965.

39. HIBAC Minutes, III: 2, December 18, 1965, p. 23.

40. Interview with former PHS economist. This official recalled a "philosophical" difference between PHS and BHI personnel on the use of Medicare funds to support hospitals. For BHI's position, see the next section of this chapter.

41. Interview with consultant to SSA.

42. For the impact of insurance on consumer preferences and hospital expenditures, see Martin S. Feldstein, *The Rising Cost of Hospital Care*, U.S. Department of Health, Education, and Welfare (Washington, D.C.: Information Resources Press, 1971).

43. See Clark C. Havighurst, "Regulation of Health Facilities and Services by 'Certificate of Need,'" *Virginia Law Review* 59 (1973): 1156-60.

44. BHI interpretation of its responsibilities, November 16, 1965, draft of "Principles for Specific Reimbursement Costs," pp. 8-9 in HIBAC Agenda Book, December 17-19, 1965.

"Historically, depreciation has not always been allowed as an element of cost, partly because it does not represent any outlay or expenditure of cash in the accounting periods after the period in which the asset was acquired. However, recognition of depreciation as an element of cost is not an issue here. The Committee reports state that reasonable costs shall include 'appropriate treatment of depreciation on buildings and equipment (taking into account such factors as the effect of Hill-Burton construction grants and practices with respect to funding).' We interpret this to be an expression of Congressional intent that depreciation shall be included in costs but that the Administration (SSA) must determine the details of what is appropriate, including the question of funding of depreciation on facilities constructed with Hill-Burton funds."

45. "Basis for Depreciation," December 15, 1965, pp. 1-2, HIBAC Agenda Book, December 17-19, 1965.

46. Ibid., "Principles for Specific Reimbursement Costs," November 16, 1965, p. 11 and "Method for Allocation of Depreciation," December 15, 1965, both in HIBAC Agenda Book, December 17-19, 1965.

47. See n. 44 above.

48. "Depreciation on Hill-Burton Assets," December 13, 1965, HIBAC Agenda Book, December 17-19, 1965.

49. Ibid.

50. Ibid.

51. "Imputed Interest," HIBAC Agenda Book, December 17-19, 1965.

52. Ibid., p. 4.

53. Ibid., p. 5.

54. Ibid., pp. 5-6. While BHI officials recognized faults in Hill-Burton financing, they nevertheless believed that the program provided for "allocation of priorities, construction standards, etc. [that] have had a salutary effect upon equitable geographical distribution of hospital beds and quality in construction."

55. The HIBAC minutes in the winter of 1965-66 reveal this as the only issue to arouse serious controversy in the council's consideration of Medicare regulations. Herman Somers, who attended the HIBAC meetings, recalled that the issue "virtually stalemated" the Council. Somers and Somers, *Medicare and the Hospitals*, p. 179.

56. See HIBAC minutes, V:1, January 28, 1966, pp. 17ff. Memorandum from Robert J. Myers, Chief Actuary, on actuarial and financial effects of making payments of imputed interest on capital under HI program; and "Considerations Involved in Determining the Proper Rate of Interest to Hospitals for the Cost of 'Equity' Capital," January 22, 1966, both in HIBAC Agenda Book, January 28-30, 1966.

57. Interview with former BHI official.

58. "Considerations Involved in Determining the Proper Rate of Interest," January 22, 1966.

59. Interview with former BHI official.

60. "Increasing the Availability of Health Facilities and Personnel." Appended to HIBAC minutes, IV, January 7-8, 1966.

61. Ibid.

62. Ibid.

63. Interviews with officials and observers.

64. Interview.

65. Interview with participants. An observer recalls that the council preferred consensus to a formal vote; thus, positions were not recorded. SSA Chief Actuary Robert Myers told the council that had he been aware of the possibility of paying imputed interest, he would have recommended to Congress a 0.1 percent increase in the payroll tax to finance it. HIBAC minutes, V:1, January 28, 1966, p. 17.

66. HIBAC minutes, V:1, January 28, 1966, p. 19.

67. Ibid., and HIBAC minutes, V:2, January 29, 1966, p. 30.

68. Letter from Kermit Gordon, Chairman of HIBAC to the Honorable John W. Gardner, Secretary of Health, Education, and Welfare, February 9, 1966, Appendix C to HIBAC minutes, V, January 28-30, 1966.

69. Ibid.

70. Interview with BHI official.

71. HIBAC minutes, V:2, January 29, 1966, p. 27. This cost estimate differs from later SSA statements on the cost of its reimbursement principles.

72. HIBAC decision, minutes, V:2, January 29, 1966, pp. 24–25. The proposal at the previous meeting had restricted advance payments to situations where necessity was demonstrated.

73. Ibid., and Commissioner Ball's testimony in U.S., Senate, Committee on Finance, *Reimbursement Guidelines for Medicare, Hearing Before the Committee on Finance*, 89th Cong., 2d sess., May 25, 1966, p. 47. In its initial recommendation BHI had rejected provider representatives' proposals to relate depreciation allocation to amortization periods. BHI felt that approach would have limited application and the straight-line depreciation would be more consistent with asset use. "Methods for Allocation of Depreciation," December 15, 1965, and "Principles for Specific Reimbursement Costs," November 19, 1965, p. 11, both in HIBAC Agenda Book, December 17–19, 1965.

74. Robert Myers explained the yield of historical cost depreciation on a straight-line and accelerated basis to HIBAC:

It is the contention of the memorandum that the historical depreciation method . . . yields *more* favorable results to hospitals than mere replacement of the object at the end of the lifetime period at the anticipated higher prices then prevailing than were in effect at the beginning of the period.

The basic reason why this is so arises from the effect of the accruing interest possible on the annual depreciation payment amounts. Such interest is, in actuality, present even if there is not separate funding and investment of the depreciation payment amounts. If such amounts are used to pay off existing debts, then the interest saved on the debt is, in reality, interest accruing on the ledger asset represented by the reduction in debt. If such amounts are used to purchase new objects, then the value of these assets, plus the depreciation amounts, and interest saved by not borrowing to buy them are properly a depreciation reserve and accumulating interest thereon, even though this is a ledger asset.

Assuming a 4 percent interest earned or creditable on a depreciation payments reserve, Myers estimated that reserve at the end of twenty years as a percentage of original cost: on a straight-line basis, 152 percent; on the accelerated double declining balance basis, 163 percent; and on the accelerated proportional basis, 171 percent. Myers noted the excess over original costs, adding his view that the excess was "more than enough to meet the current replacement cost," considering a rise in the general price level of 1-1.5 percent per year and under some circumstances, expansion to meet population growth of about 1.5 percent per year. Myers questioned even the allowance of accelerated depreciation

. . . since even the straight-line one is so advantageous to hospitals when interest effects are considered (as they properly must be). The fact that income-tax provisions allow these methods (and thus a real 'break' for taxpayers) is irrelevant because under the HI program the principle is one of 'reasonable cost' and not 'tax advantages.'

(Memorandum dated January 24, 1966. Subject: Historical Cost Depreciation with Straight-line or Accelerated Method is More than Current Replacement Cost. HIBAC Agenda Book, January 28–30, 1966.)

75. HIBAC minutes, IV:2, January 8, 1966, pp. 18–21. BHI Deputy Director Howard Bost informed the council that this option could be restricted to assets without records or applied to all assets acquired before 1966. The council requested the development of safeguards against abuse, and opted for the latter. Ball explained this decision to the Senate Finance Committee as intended "to avoid the possibility that an institution might be penalized for having good books." Committee on Finance, *Reimbursement Guidelines for Medicare*, p. 47.

76. Commissioner Ball in Committee on Finance, *Reimbursement Guidelines for Medicare*, p. 47.

77. HIBAC discussion, minutes, II, November 21, 1965, p. 15.

78. See in particular HIBAC minutes, III:2, December 18, 1965, pp. 20–25. At the previous meeting "A suggestion that one way of avoiding such problems would be to make the payments for depreciation to a central community fund was considered impractical by several members of the Council because hospitals generally would not accept such a suggestion." HIBAC minutes, II, November 21, 1965, p. 15.

79. HIBAC minutes, VIII:1, April 30, 1966, p. 9.

80. Interview with BHI official and Commissioner Ball in Committee on Finance, *Reimbursement Guidelines for Medicare*, p. 59.

81. Interview with former BHI official. This official explained that hospitals were then using these funds to cover charity cases, which Medicare did not consider an allowable cost.

82. In response to the Senate Finance Committee staff critique of their decision, SSA also argued that (1) compulsory funding for proprietary institutions might be considered depriving them of their own capital; (2) it might similarly interfere with state and local prerogatives to create or cease to create public facilities; and (3) because few localities had effective planning organizations, a funding-with-planning requirement would tie up funds for much of the hospital system while the planning network was brought into existence. Committee on Finance, *Reimbursement Guidelines for Medicare*, p. 102.

83. For comments on the inconsistency of this argument with the justification of depreciation as a contribution to future capital needs, see Somers and Somers, *Medicare and the Hospitals*, pp. 175–77.

84. HIBAC minutes, VIII:1, April 30, 1966, p. 9. The General Accounting Office questioned the desirability of providing this incentive to fund when there was no contractual commitment or guarantee that the funds would be used for the intended purpose, that is, investment in capital. ("Review of Proposed Principles of Reimbursement for Provider Costs under Public Law 89–97," Department

of Health, Education, and Welfare, Social Security Administration, Report to the Committee on Finance, U.S. Senate, by the Comptroller General of the United States, appendix A to Committee on Finance, *Reimbursement Guidelines for Medicare*, pp. 176–77.)

In response BHI changed its payment rules to specify that unless depreciation funds were used for capital purposes related to patient care, interest earned on them would be deducted from allowable costs in determining reimbursement. "Principles of Reimbursement for Provider Costs," 20 C.F.R. Sec. 405.419; and HIBAC minutes, IX:1, June 3, 1966, p. 8.

85. A former AHA official disagreed, but contemporary accounts support this SSA official's account. Also see Somers and Somers, *Medicare and the Hospitals*, p. 180.

86. "Hospitals Gain Last Minute Concessions in Medicare Reimbursement Principles Announced in Los Angeles," reprinted from *Modern Hospital*, May 1966, as appendix C to Committee on Finance, *Reimbursement Guidelines for Medicare*, p. 191, reprinted with permission.

87. Final arrangements reported in "Reimbursement under Medicare," reprinted from *Hospitals, J.A.H.A.*, May 16, 1966, reprinted as appendix D in Committee on Finance, *Reimbursement Guidelines for Medicare*, p. 195.

88. Interview with BHI official.

89. Letter from Kenneth Williamson, associate director, AHA, to Senator Russell B. Long, chairman, Senate Finance Committee, appendix B to Committee on Finance, *Reimbursement Guidelines for Medicare*, p. 186.

90. HIBAC minutes, VIII:1, April 30, 1966, p. 7. Quote is of a summary, not verbatim.

91. See Ball's explanation of reimbursement principles, Committee on Finance, *Reimbursement Guidelines for Medicare*, especially p. 48; Somers and Somers, *Medicare and the Hospitals*, pp. 180–81. Emphasis later shifted further to "various elements not specifically recognized in the formula or not precisely measured." Ball, Committee on Finance, *Reimbursement Guidelines for Medicare*, p. 56. See n. 118 below.

92. HIBAC minutes, VIII:1, April 30, 1966, p. 7.

93. Interviews with officials.

94. Interview with senior SSA official.

95. Interview with BHI official.

96. "Hospitals Gain Last Minute Concessions," appendix C to Committee on Finance, *Reimbursement Guidelines for Medicare*, p. 192.

97. Resolution dated May 21, 1966, appended to letter from Kenneth Williamson to Senator Long, appendix B to Committee on Finance, *Reimbursement Guidelines for Medicare*, p. 188.

98. Press release dated May 4, 1966, appendix 1 to Staff Report on Proposed Medicare Reimbursement Formula in Committee on Finance, *Reimbursement Guidelines for Medicare*, p. 39.

99. Committee on Finance, *Reimbursement Guidelines for Medicare*, pp. 52–53.

100. Ibid. pp. 118 and 120-22.

101. Ibid., p. 111.

102. See "Proposed Medicare Reimbursement Formula," Ibid. The Committee staff also objected to two other aspects of the reimbursement principles: (1) the advance payment of working capital and (2) the absence of a return on equity for proprietary institutions. With regard to depreciation, the staff argued:

The legislative history and statute indicate that the Medicare program is a cost reimbursement program, and where Federal or State tax revenues are involved, we don't consider that to be a cost to the hospital.

We look on those grants as other than a cost—as a non-cost. Since the hospital hasn't incurred a cost, it is difficult for us to understand why the hospital should be granted an allowance for depreciation on that public money.

Now, this committee, at least for 12 years, has followed the practice in the tax laws of not allowing depreciation on contributed property, or on property that is purchased with contributions.

We look on the Federal grant or even the State grant as contributed property, and under the tax law this committee would frown if depreciation were allowed on it.

Yet the medicare reimbursement guidelines allow for depreciation on those assets paid for with public money. "Proposed Medicare Reimbursement Formula," p. 99.

103. Ibid. See, for example, pp. 111-12. Senator Anderson attributed the term "sweetener" to the AHA.

104. Ibid. See, for example, p. 108.

105. Ibid. See, for example, pp. 59, 70, 112-16.

106. Ibid.

107. Ibid., pp. 59, 102, 113, and 115-16.

108. Ibid., p. 113.

109. Ibid., pp. 110-11.

110. Ibid., p. 111.

111. Ibid., p. 117.

112. Ibid., p. 117.

113. Ibid., p. 117.

114. Ibid., pp. 52-53, Senator Abraham Ribicoff (D-Connecticut): "In other words you have made tentative agreements with all institutions. Now we come in after you have made tentative agreements. This goes into effect July 1, and here it is almost the end of May. . . . Now, you have the embarrassing situation, if you change it, you probably cause almost a revolution and confusion within weeks before the plan goes into effect." Page 108, Senator Douglas: "But with the shortage of time, personally, Mr. Chairman, I don't think we should tear this system up by the roots at the last minute." See also p. 122.

115. Ibid., pp. 59-60.

116. Interview.

117. As minor changes, SSA had already lowered the ceiling on the 2 percent plus factor by excluding Hill-Burton assets from net equity, thereby eliminating a discrepancy between proprietary and nonprofit hospitals; had renamed "advance" payments "current" payments; and responded to the GAO by specifying that unless depreciation funds were used for capital purposes related to patient care, interest earned on them would be deducted from allowable costs in reimbursement. "Principles of Reimbursement for Provider Costs," 20 C.F.R. Sec. 405.419; and HIBAC Minutes IX:1, June 3, 1966, p. 8.

118. HIBAC considered a distinction between nonprofit and proprietary hospitals for reimbursement purposes, particularly after they agreed not to pay imputed interest. In July 1965, they decided to recommended that reimbursement to proprietary institutions include a reasonable return on equity, accompanied by straight-line depreciation and a possible reduction in the 2 percent plus factor. (HIBAC minutes, X:2, July 13, 1966, pp. 28-32) Senator Long supported payment of a profit to proprietaries in the May hearings (Committee on Finance, *Reimbursement Guidelines for Medicare*, p. 58). SSA and HEW resisted these pressures. Interviews suggest that their decision to treat all hospitals alike was a product of two factors: (1) the belief that a financial advantage to proprietary hospitals was inconsistent with national policy and the general view in the field that nonprofits were superior institutions; and (2) the general principle that treating some institutions better than others might be "inequitable." The 2 percent plus was intended to satisfy everybody's demand for a "return" (See, for example, Commissioner Ball in Committee on Finance, *Reimbursement Guidelines for Medicare*, p. 56, and HIBAC discussion, X:2, July 13, 1966, pp. 28-32).

The American Nursing Home Association (ANHA) launched a successful campaign to have Congress override this decision (See Somers and Somers, *Medicare and the Hospitals*, p. 183, and appendix A to ANHA testimony in U.S., Congress, Senate, Committee on Finance, *Social Security Amendments of 1970, Hearings before the Committee on Finance on H.R. 17550*, 91st Cong., 2d sess., 1970, pp. 695 ff). Officials described their opposition to this amendment on policy and administrative grounds. In conference they were able to lower the base for calculating the return from asset value to equity and put a ceiling on the rate. A former BHI official recalled these changes as a "coup." "The proprietaries didn't know what they didn't have until they didn't have it" (Interview).

Because the amendment also reduced the plus factor for proprietaries to 1.5 percent, it further shifted the rationale for the plus factor from a "return on equity" to a payment for unmeasurable costs (See Somers and Somers, *Medicare and the Hospitals*, pp. 183-85).

Paying the Hospitals: Maintaining the Bargain

The 1966 rules for Medicare reimbursement could have been only a beginning for Medicare payment policy, subject to reevaluation and change in the light of experience. That experience turned out markedly favorable to the hospitals.

It was widely feared by hospitals that the Medicare program would result in losses to hospital operations. In fact, hospital revenues have risen slightly faster than expenses since the introduction of Medicare, and a fairly substantial increase in hospital net incomes has resulted. Net incomes of community hospitals went from $198 million in fiscal 1966 to $270 million in fiscal year 1968 . . . Cash flows of community hospitals (net incomes plus depreciation expenses) also rose considerably—from $625 million in 1966 to $1.0 billion in 1968.[1]

As net income increased, so did hospital expenditures.

Expenses per patient day in community hospitals increased at an annual rate of 12.2 percent in the first two years of the Medicare program, compared with 6.8 percent in the pre-Medicare period. Although this was a time of accelerating price inflation in the economy as a whole, all of the increase in hospital costs cannot be attributed to that source. The consumer price index rose at an annual rate of 3.5 [percent] during the period.[2]

Hospitals took advantage of expanded revenues "to raise the 'quality' of hospital care as perceived by hospital decision-makers—that is, to increase the quantities of inputs (labor and equipment) used to provide a day of hospital care."[3] As Karen Davis has explained it:

Hospitals "break even," not by keeping their prices down to minimum cost levels, but by increasing their costs to equal the maximum revenue which they are able to collect without adversely affecting hospital utilization.[4]

This behavior was not new with Medicare; it was typical of hospitals' responses to increases in consumer purchasing power, whether financed by public or private insurance or by rising incomes. But following the enactment of Medicare, and, at the same time, Medicaid to finance medical services for the poor, hospitals increased their expenditures and charges more rapidly than ever before.[5]

SSA had contributed to this phenomenon with its liberal 1965–1966 decisions on hospital reimbursement, but they did not necessarily have to continue this policy thereafter. Had they changed their political strategy from balancing to cost-effectiveness after 1966, they might have responded to Medicare's impact with a reconsideration of both their initial concessions and cost reimbursement as a whole.

In fact, however, assessments of political balance continued to shape SSA's payment policy and entrenched the 1966 reimbursement rules. SSA's policy judgments reveal implicit and explicit calculations of the political and administrative costs of change versus the benefits of the status quo. Where they felt political pressure, the agency made an effort to appear responsive; where they did not, they resisted proposals for change. Their strategy was to avoid adjustments in reimbursement that might provoke conflict with the hospitals or rekindle their payment demands. By maintaining the status quo, SSA balanced the interests of their potential antagonists, the hospitals and the Congress, and kept their working relationship with the hospitals on an even keel. The following account of SSA's policies toward prepaid group practices, reimbursement experiments, and program administration illustrates the way SSA resisted and avoided disruption of its 1966 arrangements.

Paying Group Practice Prepayment Plans

Despite controversy, Medicare administrators fulfilled their promise that the hospitals would be paid according to principles of their own making. But that reimbursement did not suit all the providers that Medicare had to pay. It was particularly unsuitable for Group Practice Prepayment Plans (GPPPs), organizations of physicians who operate quite differently from most of the nation's physicians and hospitals. GPPPs contract to provide their members whatever medical care they need in return for fixed monthly payments (advance capitation). Plan physicians are not paid a fee for each service they render, but rather a fixed amount per patient (capitation), a salary, or a share of plan income. Because of this financial structure, GPPPs' net income does not increase with the volume of services delivered, unlike most hospitals and physicians. On the contrary, GPPP net income is higher when it delivers fewer services. GPPP members tend to use hospitals far less frequently than the rest of the population, a result frequently attributed to the incentives of the payment system. As a result of these savings, GPPPs can generally offer consumers more comprehensive coverage than third-party insurance for approximately the same monthly payment.[6]

The retroactive cost reimbursement Medicare used for hospitals and its fee-for-service reimbursement for physicians would completely disrupt these operations. Paying retroactively for services actually delivered would remove GPPP incentives for efficient use of medical services; eliminate the difference between capitation and cost with which they financed additional services; and so disrupt their management, accounting, and budgeting operations. In essence, it would turn GPPPs into fee-for-service operations for their Medicare members.

Because of these problems, GPPP reimbursement posed a choice for Medicare administrators. If they had pursued a cost-effectiveness strategy, they would have investigated the advantages of GPPPs and might have used the payment system to encourage their development. With a balancing strategy, these advantages would have been irrelevant and SSA would have paid for care in GPPPs according to the dictates of political pressure. Because GPPPs were few in number and had little political backing, SSA would probably have paid them the same way they paid for care everywhere else. In fact SSA *did* base its payment to GPPPs on the principles they had already developed for most hospitals and physicians, with few adjustments to fit GPPP needs. Officials thereby averted the political and administrative costs of interfering with the interests and arrangements of the medical care establishment—hospitals, physicians, and insurers. At the same time, officials perceived few if any benefits to accommodating GPPPs. The following account illustrates how this calculation both explicitly and implicitly influenced Medicare policy.

GPPPs were concerned about their reimbursement even before the Medicare law was enacted. They tried to get specific authorization for capitation in the 1965 Medicare law, but were reportedly opposed by Wilbur Cohen.[7] While Cohen staunchly supported prepaid group practice, a former GPPP lobbyist explained, he felt that a specific legislative provision would antagonize the American Medical Association, which had bitterly opposed GPPP development over the years. Cohen's alternative was general legislative language that administrators could interpret favorably to GPPPs after the law had passed.[8] In the end the legislative record had both specific and general provisions for prepayment plans. Provisions on physician payment specifically allowed cost rather than charge reimbursement for prepayment plans,[9] and the committee reports called special attention to the advantages of prepayment:

In establishing the complementary [hospital and physician] plans for medical care for the aged in this bill, no special recognition is being given to the lower rate of hospital utilization which might be experienced by aged persons under comprehensive health care plans. However, it is not the intention of your committee by this action to adversely affect those organizations which provide and operate comprehensive health care services. On the other hand, it is the hope of your committee that the development of comprehensive health care plans be encouraged.[10]

When it came time to make payment rules, however, the specific language proved inadequate and the favorable interpretation failed to materialize. BHI did not look to GPPP past practices and develop reimbursement to suit them, as they had with the hospitals. Instead they started with the reimbursement methods they had developed for the bulk of the nation's providers and tried to make them fit GPPPs. They were willing to tinker with their reimbursement formulas, but not to abandon them in favor of the advance capitation of prepayment.

Accordingly, BHI interpreted the law as requiring retroactive cost-based reimbursement, limited to services the plans actually provided to beneficiaries, and refused to allow plans to control the use and costs of services arranged rather than provided directly for their members. More specifically, member beneficiaries and providers used by but not part of the plan would not be required to receive services or reimbursement through the plan. Furthermore, the law was interpreted to require that hospital reimbursement be paid directly to the hospital.[11]

Dissatisfied, the plans protested, seeking advance capitation for services made available, rather than provided, and maintenance of total control over the payment and delivery of care to their members.[12] Their position was perhaps most cogently stated to HIBAC by Glenn Wilson, a GPPP administrator:

The Social Security Administration has properly insured that there will be no interference in the traditional solo practice fee-for-service provision of health care. Such has not been the case in the relationship between the Social Security Administration and the prepaid group practice plans. . . . The application of P.L. 89–97 has produced significant organizational disadvantages for prepaid group practice plans. . . .

Capitation has historically been defined by the prepaid group practice plans as the amount of money required per person to make available covered services to a group of eligible persons for a specified time.

What is being applied by SSA is not capitation in any real sense of the word. It is true that it is called capitation but individual services must then be reported and SSA has insisted that at the end of a given period adjustments will be made retroactively to reflect the services actually provided. The essence of group practice is ease of referral and consultation among various medical disciplines. A personal physician may consult a surgeon simply by going down the hall and securing necessary advice. It is impossible to record all such consultations in a group practice without strangling paper work. In solo practice such consultations are clearly two visits. Group practice plans will almost certainly miss reporting many such consultations. . . .[13]

In materials presented to HIBAC, Wilson stressed the need for plan control of all services provided members:

SSA does not understand that prepaid group practice plans assume the responsibility for all the medical services a member of the plan may require whether or not the member is covered or uncovered by the plan, whether or not the service is provided by a physician associated with the plan. This obligation to arrange whatever medical care is needed regardless of the time of day or the day of the year is essential for the continuity of care regardless of whether a member is out of the area, has an in-area emergency or is referred to an out-of-plan specialist. It is the obligation of the health plan to insure that the services are of high quality and do not duplicate previous care.[14]

As summarized by Dr. Lorin Kerr, president of the plans' trade association, the Group Health Association of America (GHAA):

The reimbursement of group practice plans under Medicare is fragmented and complex, with the result that plans are losing control over services they normally provide to their non-Medicare enrollees, and beneficiaries are in some cases required to pay out cash and be reimbursed by a cumbersome process for services that other enrollees receive without such charges.[15]

Other effects of BHI policy that the plans did not emphasize included: (1) the elimination of existing financial incentives,[16] and (2) the disruption of plan arrangements by the imposition between plan and out-of-plan providers of intermediaries, which, generally closely tied to fee-for-service medicine, the plans may have felt they could not trust.[17]

The GPPPs proposed that Medicare pay them advance capitation (without retroactive adjustment) for services made available rather than actually provided. To obtain responsibility and authority to arrange and pay for all services provided their members while conforming to BHI's interpretation of the law, they proposed that they be designated carriers or intermediaries. Although the plans preferred a single capitation payment to cover both hospital and physician services, they were willing to accept separate payment consistent with the division of the Medicare program into hospital and physician services.[18]

BHI continued to find these arrangements in conflict with the law. Their reasoning on the following issues reflected both their unwillingness to make arrangements for GPPPs that conflicted with their agreements with the prevailing medical care establishment, and the priority they gave to the privileges of that establishment. First, BHI rejected capitation on the grounds that it was underwriting, or taking financial risk for benefit payments.[19] Insurers had sought this privilege in the Medicare law, and Congress and Medicare architects had turned them down.[20] Administrators would not now grant it to someone else.

Second, despite the fact that membership in plans was voluntary and that plans were controlling out-of-plan services before Medicare, BHI rejected Medicare conformity to that practice as a violation of the "rights of beneficiaries, physicians and providers."

Under the program as enacted, the Medicare beneficiary who is a member of a group practice prepayment plan is provided his basic health insurance protection under a national insurance system that will cover him for services provided to him without regard to whether or not the plan provides, arranges or is otherwise involved in the provision of services. The beneficiary may, therefore, claim reimbursement for medical services covered by the Medicare program whether or not they are provided under a group practice prepayment plan of which he is a member. The reasonable charge of a nonplan physician rendering covered medical services to a beneficiary who is a member of a group practice prepayment plan will, therefore, provide the base for reimbursement whether or not it is established by agreement with the plan. And even if the law did not require—as it does—direct reimbursement of providers for the cost of services covered under Part A, the beneficiary would have the right to seek covered services in any participating facility, without regard to whether or not the facility had an arrangement with his plan, and the participating facility would have the right to seek reimbursement for these services, just as it would for services to any other beneficiary of the program. We do not believe that it is possible under the law to adopt administrative procedures, or that it would be desirable to amend the law to allow the adoption of administrative procedures, that would dilute these rights of beneficiaries, physicians and providers.[21]

Third, BHI ruled that the plans could not be intermediaries for their members. BHI had resisted insurance companies' efforts to act as the intermediaries or carriers for their private beneficiaries wherever they received care, and instead appointed a fiscal agent for each institution or physician. In this way, a former BHI official explained, the fiscal agent could exercise some sort of control over services. Having insisted to insurance companies that there could only be one intermediary per hospital, BHI did not want to reverse itself for GPPPs,[22] even though it would enhance fiscal control. BHI explained this decision in terms of administrative convenience.

It must also be recognized that the administration of the medicare program is, by virtue of the interrelationships that it requires between Federal and State agencies, providers, intermediaries, carriers, physicians and beneficiaries, already quite complex. Under such conditions, administrative feasibility must be a major consideration in weighing any policy or proposed policy. We do not believe that it would be administratively feasible to enter into arrangements that would require providers to deal with a multiplicity of intermediaries or require physicians to deal with a multiplicity of carriers.[23]

On the grounds that GPPPs were "providers," BHI and HEW's General Counsel also argued that designating GPPPs intermediaries of carriers would constitute a conflict of interest. The plans' response emphasizes the difference in BHI's treatment of GPPPs as compared with conventional institutions:

If the prepaid group practice plans have a conflict of interest in being carriers and providers, then certainly Blue Cross plans in most sections of the country are already involved in this conflict of interest. In most instances, Blue Cross Boards are, by statute, required to be representatives *of the hospitals*. In Ohio the majority of the Board of Directors of Blue Cross, by law, must be hospitals. SSA has refused to acknowledge in discussions the Blue Cross situation. They continue to repeat that prepaid group practice plans can't be carriers because of the conflict of interest. We insist that these decisions are inconsistent and that either prepaid group practice plans can be carriers or Blue Cross cannot be carriers.[24]

These arguments persuaded neither HIBAC nor BHI. Although HIBAC responded to a GPPP presentation by instructing BHI "to facilitate GPPP operations,"[25] a former council member associated with GPPPs described his fellow members as generally unsupportive of the plans' position. Physician members, he recalled, were adamantly opposed to developing special arrangements for

GPPPs. This member paraphrased the predominant viewpoint: if GPPPs were "as good as they were cracked up to be," there was no reason to give them special treatment.[26] BHI would not accede to the GPPPs' primary demands, but did respond to their arguments with some administrative changes. Among them was an arrangement whereby a member could submit bills for nonplan services to the plans, and the plan could pay them and be reimbursed. This would respond to some of the problems of members' inconvenience cited by the plans but, as BHI recognized, not the major fiscal and organizational ones. Also, all GPPPs were permitted to deal directly with SSA rather than through carriers on physician payment, an arrangement previously restricted to those choosing cost rather than charge reimbursement. And, seemingly in contradiction of the conflict of interest argument—but consistent with noninterference with out-of-plan providers—GPPPs that owned their own hospitals were allowed to serve as intermediaries for them.[27]

In making these and other changes, BHI officials thought they were being as responsive to GPPPs as the law would allow. Asked to explain their decision, officials recalled: "We did all we could for them under the law."[28] But Medicare administrators had interpreted the law with remarkable ingenuity when it came to hospital reimbursement. Why would they not do the same for GPPPs? Part of the answer was clearly BHI's overwhelming involvement in reimbursement for the conventional system. A former GPPP representative attributed much of BHI's behavior to their preoccupation with the vast majority of medical care providers, absorption in the traditional insurance approach, and unfamiliarity with prepaid group practice. He described the agency's failure to respond to GPPPs as an "error of omission."[29]

But what was and was not omitted in Medicare payment policy suggests the importance in BHI's decisions of political as well as administrative concerns. In contrast to the hospitals, whose satisfaction Medicare officials found essential, GPPPs were a small number of providers whose cooperation with the program was relatively inconsequential. Medicare did not need them; they needed Medicare. To administrators developing a reimbursement system for all sorts of medical care institutions, GPPPs appeared one more interest group seeking all they could get.[30] Unlike the nation's hospitals, the GPPPs lacked the support of the medical establishment. Their demands would interfere with the "rights" of that establishment and could provoke it to cause administrators trouble. SSA had no reason to incur these costs; accommodation of GPPPs was a demand they could withstand.

Reimbursement Experimentation

As soon as Medicare went into operation, medical cost inflation began to receive public attention. Before 1966, the medical price index rose at an annual rate of

2.5 percent; the 1966 index rose 6.6 percent. Hospital charges had risen 6.0 percent per year between 1960 and 1965; in 1966 they increased 16.5 percent.[31] The administration recognized the problem, but was still primarily concerned with expanding health insurance protection. In 1967 they proposed legislation to include in Medicare the disabled beneficiaries of Social Security.[32] At the same time they dealt with costs by convening conferences[33] and commissioning reports.[34] From these came two recommendations for Medicare reimbursement that the administration included in legislative proposals: (1) making depreciation reimbursement contingent on funding and approval of capital expenditures by state planning agencies; and (2) including incentives for efficiency in the reimbursement formula. The planning requirement followed directly from the Senate Finance Committee's reaction to the initial reimbursement regulations.[35] Opposed by the hospitals, Blue Cross–Blue Shield, and the largest prepaid group practice plan, the proposal was defeated in the House, passed in modified form by the Senate, and dropped in conference.[36] Thus Congress endorsed SSA's initial decision on planning and reimbursement.

The Congress did enact another amendment to reimbursement that SSA proposed. The multitude of health cost conferences and reports criticized cost reimbursement on the grounds that it offered institutions no incentives for efficient delivery of health services. In other words, a hospital being reimbursed for costs had no reason to minimize those costs. A clamor arose in health circles for the incorporation of incentives in Medicare reimbursement.[37] In response SSA proposed and Congress authorized experimentation with alternatives to cost reimbursement that offered institutions incentives for efficiency.[38]

With a cost-effectiveness strategy, SSA might have used the clamor and the legislative authority to evaluate its reimbursement principles and explore new alternatives. In fact, SSA was not reconsidering its earlier decisions in 1967 and 1968. Although they had promised the hospitals, HIBAC, and the Senate Finance Committee a prompt review of their reimbursement policy,[39] that promise was intended primarily to reassure those who thought Medicare would pay hospitals too little. To paraphrase one BHI official: "The promise to review was a concession to the hospitals, i.e., we'd change if we'd been too cheap. We hadn't been, so there was no review."[40] The absence of any pressure within or from HIBAC to reconsider capital reimbursement in 1967 and 1968 was striking.[41] As one member explained, rising costs sent imputed interest "out the window."[42] Neither the Congress nor the administration viewed the experimentation amendment as a comprehensive reevaluation of Medicare. Instead, as SSA's handling of experimentation reveals, it was a means of responding to external criticism of reimbursement policy without making policy changes.

The first indication of this intent was the attitude of officials responsible for reimbursement experiments. Far from sharing the health field's enthusiasm for incentive reimbursement, Irwin Wolkstein, then assistant director of the Bureau of Health Insurance, expressed considerable skepticism about its impact:

It should be understood that the potential for economy through financial rewards and deterrents is limited. There are many motivations and factors in a complex hospital other than maximizing net operating income from third parties. For one thing, contributions from the community at large, as from specific donors, may sometimes be induced by almost the opposite of economy of operation. The success of a hospital in its administration may be measured not merely by hospital efficiency but also by the completeness of hospital facilities, the fame of its staff, and the wealth of its patients. None of these is necessarily highly correlated with efficiency. . . .[43]

Writing in 1969, Wolkstein expanded on the multiplicity of incentives within a hospital:

Hospital administrators and other health service managers are as a group well intentioned in avoiding waste and do so sometimes to the extent of financial disadvantage of their institutions. However, health service managers have other objectives besides saving money. First, minimizing the risk of an error that may result in dismissal may be preferable to maximizing the likelihood of cost reduction. Second, administrators generally seek to spend funds in ways that will advance their organizations. The success of and the incomes of hospital managers are closely tied to the success of the institutions that employ them. . . .

The point here is that there are a large number of incentives brought to bear in health care, some leading to and others leading away from higher costs. Some of the pressures that lead to ineffective practices will not be easily overcome. For one thing, a physician's livelihood depends on his hospital having the facilities that help him care for patients and he will not be satisfied if the demands can only be met in some other hospital by some other physician. . . . Pressure for duplication and an excess of capacity in hospitals will be strong so long as the excesses are advantageous to doctors and the cost of the excess falls only indirectly on patients through the premiums and taxes they pay.[44]

In the context of these incentives, a hospital facing a choice between full cost reimbursement and a share in any savings below a target would be unlikely to choose the latter. In nonprofit institutions, funds are applied to hospital expenses, not individual incomes. Thus with cost reimbursement the hospital could get more of what it wanted than with the incentive reward. An institution that wants to spend money has no financial reason to prefer saving money to spend it over simply spending money and receiving full cost reimbursement. Although some might participate for other reasons, a study by Bauer and Densen suggests the decidedly limited appeal of such an approach:

For example, in 1970 before Rhode Island launched its statewide prospective budgeting system, Blue Cross and the largest hospital in the state cooperated in a pilot demonstration of the incentive plan. The hospital reduced a proposed $38 million budget for 1970–1971 by almost $1 million during the course of the budget review and target rate negotiations, and then managed to spend $250,000 less than the final budget figure. In return it got an incentive payment of $25,000. It was an impressive achievement by a dedicated administrator. But over the years and in more typical hospitals is the prospect of a reward of this size likely to move an institution to forego the benefits it presumably believes would flow from an extra million dollars?[45]

BHI officials asked precisely this question. SSA and HEW called the problem of voluntary participation to congressional attention shortly after the amendment was passed,[46] but Congress never acted. A BHI memorandum reports that in 1969's deliberations, the Ways and Means Committee noted

the difficulty of justifying the use of one area over another on a compulsory basis, and the absence of an effective alternative course of action for a provider that did not want to participate.[47]

Although a congressional participant attributed the committee's rejection of compulsory participation to their belief that voluntarism was not the problem with the experimental program,[48] an administration participant felt that the congressmen's attitude was "Not in my district."[49] Whether a question of equity, necessity, or politics, no action was taken.

With little confidence in its usefulness, experimentation was a low priority for BHI.[50] The most positive description of officials' attitudes toward incentive reimbursement was that they felt it should at least be tried.[51] The "trial" produced five experiments by 1972.[52] At that time BHI explained to HIBAC "why hundreds of proposals submitted under the 1967 legislation have resulted in only five experiments."[53] Part of the explanation[54] was SSA's research strategy, a second indication of the program's purpose. BHI did not develop formal and specific Requests for Proposals, with which government usually solicits private research. Instead, they prepared general guidelines and waited for specific experimental proposals from the outside. An official explained: "We were dealing with AHA, the intermediaries, the Health Insurance Association of America—they all have Research and Development units; we expected proposals from them."[55] It might be said tht BHI's attitude was: If you've got such good ideas, where are they? BHI themselves later described their strategy similarly, though more eloquently, as

designed to tap the vast reservoir of ideas for reimbursement incentives believed to have been already developed by the health services industry and ready for implementation with little or no additional attention. A widescale campaign was launched to elicit submittal of a supply of unique proposals sufficient to cover the full spectrum of possibilities.[56]

That strategy was unsuccessful. As BHI later explained, the research expertise and capacity in the health care industry that they intended to rely upon did not exist. As a result, proposals were incomplete and lacked plans for data collection and evaluation.[57]

That BHI relied on external initiative was more a matter of strategy than of lack of ideas. A BHI report to HIBAC early in the experimental program suggested the following range of experimental objectives: open staffing to eliminate duplication of facilities resulting from restricted staff privileges; pooled capital, that is, testing the effects of determining and contributing to overall capital needs in a given area rather than hospital by hospital; testing the effect of encouraging GPPP expansion on the efficiency and economy of delivery of care in an area; and testing capitation in a nongroup practice setting, such as a medical foundation.[58] Interviews support the interest of at least some BHI officials in some of these ideas, particularly the first two. They never constituted a blueprint for experimentation, however, probably because BHI's interest in experimentation was limited, and because hospitals only participated in experiments that appealed to them.

In fact, BHI regarded providers' attitudes as an additional, "perhaps more serious" factor in explaining how little experimentation was undertaken.[59] BHI described this factor as "a misunderstanding of the nature of the program."

Certain organizations have seen the experimental program as a way to achieve changes in Medicare reimbursement that would improve the financial position of hospitals, i.e., changes that would tend to increase costs rather than contain or reduce them. Inclusion of bad debts and charity, and capital expense limited only by planning approval were the primary changes sought. The proposals sponsored by the Indiana and Oklahoma Hospital Associations were attempts to make all or part of the American Hospital Association Statement of Financial Requirements a part of Medicare reimbursement including provision for payment of bad debts, charity, and capital limited only by planning agency approval as needed. Either of these proposals would have been costly to the program.[60]

Interviews indicate that BHI officials saw the vast majority of experimentation proposals as "ripoffs" of the Medicare trust fund. They had tried to withstand hospital demands in 1965–1966 and were not going to give in to more demands now. Thus, while they were not committed to using Section 402 to encourage efficient hospital behavior, officials *were* committed to prohibiting providers from using it simply to obtain funds that BHI had already denied them. They therefore insisted that experimental proposals specify and provide for the measurement and evaluation of their contribution to efficiency, and rejected any proposal that would cost more than the ongoing reimbursement approach after a brief period.[61]

Experiments actually undertaken confirmed BHI's skepticism of provider interest in incentive reimbursement. As a third explanation for so little experimentation, BHI reported to HIBAC that it proved difficult in an inflationary situation in which there were also rapid changes in technology to arrive at a rate of reimbursement that appeared to hold significant promise of cost reduction and at the same time offered the provider as much safety as does full cost reimbursement. Those organizations most likely to benefit could be expected to participate in such an experiment whereas those that anticipated some adverse impact could not.[62]

Because of the possibility of loss in one approved experiment, BHI said, hospitals refused to participate and the experiment never got started.[63] Furthermore, BHI explained, other experiments were not even considered, because of the impossibility of obtaining participation.[64] Two of their five experiments did expose hospitals to possible losses, that is, posed financial risks. The Connecticut and Maryland experiments were supposed to have penalties. In the former, however, an official reported that "wherever they were applied, the hospitals quit,"[65] and in the latter, where targets were apparently "never understood," attempts to enforce them almost ended the experiment.[66]

These results suggest that SSA's skepticism was well-founded. However, their desire to prevent waste of Medicare funds made them resist potentially valuable change. General caution meant little innovation. SSA's treatment of GPPPs under Section 402 illustrates this effect. Prepayment plans received considerable attention in discussions of health cost inflation and ways to control it in 1967 and 1968. In February 1967, for example, the Gorham Report to the president on Medical Care Prices advocated encouragement of group practice, especially prepaid group practice, as a demonstrably more efficient approach to delivery of medical care.[67] The June 1967 Conference on Medical Care Costs encouraged SSA and HEW to recognize the substantial economies of prepaid group practice plans in use of hospitals, manpower, and comprehensive care. A recommendation was made that through regulation or legislation Medicare and Medicaid should reimburse these plans for all services provided on a capitation basis.[68] Congress also called special attention to GPPPs in the committee reports on Section 402.

Group practice prepayment plans that have elected to be reimbursed on a cost basis for physicians' services, and also provide hospital services, could engage in experiments under which a combined system of reimbursement could be developed for both physician and hospital services.[69]

The prepayment plans clearly thought this provision authorized the advance capitation that BHI had denied them. Major GPPPs such as Kaiser, the Health Insurance Plan (HIP) of New York, and the Community Health Association of Detroit submitted proposals to BHI for combined capitation for hospital and medical services, set in advance, and less than or equal to Medicare experience for nonmembers in the same area.[70]

Had SSA wished to encourage GPPP development by granting them advance capitation, they might have used Section 402 to do it. For GPPPs as well as hospitals, however, BHI refused to approve in an experiment what they had denied in reimbursement. According to their rules,

the experimental plan must be a plan whose premise could not be tested without some change in the application of the present cost reimbursement provision.[71]

SSA officials felt that since GPPPs were operating outside Medicare, their efficiency could be evaluated, and there was no reason to "experiment" with them in Medicare. Although Irwin Wolkstein described GPPPs as having "some of the characteristics of laboratories" for incentive reimbursement,[72] they were apparently regarded as laboratories that Medicare did not have to support.

The plans' proposals also conflicted with BHI's rule that experimental reimbursement not exceed existing reimbursement after a short period of time. Looking at an individual prepaid group practice, cost reimbursement was likely to be less than capitation reimbursement would have been.[73] By paying only for actual hospital stays, Medicare could reap the advantages of prepayment plans' lower hospital use without paying for the system associated with it.

Wolkstein of BHI challenged the connection between prepayment and lower hospital use. Rather than test capitation, Wolkstein suggested that

much more needs to be known and disclosed about the specific course which has been followed in achieving the observed rate of hospital use. The specific kinds of cases where surgery is performed less frequently in group practice than outside need to be documented. The relationship between increased outpatient service and reduced inpatient service needs to be proved; an assumption is not sufficient. Whether shorter stays occur for comparable illnesses needs to be determined; the ways in which stays are shortened need to be checked and the health results of the different patterns of care should be ascertained.[74]

To GPPPs, who wanted reimbursement consistent with their overall operation, BHI appeared overly concerned with evaluation. A plan lobbyist equated BHI's questions on "what is quality care" to "what is truth"–too philosophical to be productive.[75] BHI did engage in one experiment with a prepaid group practice, dealing with physician incentives, not capitation, and designed to cost SSA less rather than more money.[76] But they did not test their own proposition that GPPP expansion, which capitation would support, might encourage lower overall costs by competing with fee-for-service medicine.[77] In 1970 HIBAC took HEW to task for not having implemented capitation reimbursement for prepaid group practice,[78] but BHI refused to use Section 402 to demonstrate what one official described as an "old issue—that Kaiser saves money."[79]

The irony in Medicare experimentation policy and its treatment of GPPPs became apparent in 1968 Senate hearings on health care organization. A spokesman for the AFL-CIO, which, like other unions, supported prepayment plans, observed:

The whole emphasis of government programs seems to be on some completely undefined and vague "innovation" and "experimentation" in the delivery of health services. Yet prepaid group practice has shown itself to be the most effective system for providing quality medical care over the prevailing fee-for-service solo practice.[80]

The irony increased as HEW advocated GPPP expansion at the same hearings. Senator Abraham Ribicoff (D-Connecticut), who chaired the hearings, asked HEW spokesmen whether any community had organized its health services in a way that could serve as an example to the rest of the country. Dr. Philip Lee, Assistant Secretary for Health, answered "Kaiser," the largest prepaid group practice plan.[81] Wilbur Cohen, who was then secretary of HEW, followed up this observation, pointing out to Ribicoff that if Kaiser's arrangements were replicated and extended throughout the country there would be high quality care for everyone.[82] Apparently, this objective was not part of officials' perspectives on Medicare policy.

In their analysis of incentive reimbursement experimentation by public and private third-party payers, Bauer and Densen suggest that Section 402 made a valuable contribution by helping policymakers "avoid serious mistakes in designing more widespread cost control measures."[83]

We assume that the prime objectives of the SSA experiments authorized by the 1967 legislation were to identify new possibilities for using reimbursement formulas to control Medicare costs, to test the feasibility of implementing these new methods under circumstances of minimal political and financial risk, to measure their acceptability and their effectiveness, to weigh their successful application on a national scale, and thus to avoid the kinds of troubles that ensued when the "reasonable cost" formula was introduced.[84]

The evidence suggests that this assumption was an overstatement. While participants no doubt learned of the complexities of incentive reimbursement,[85] this was more a by-product than a goal of Section 402. BHI's skepticism of incentive reimbursement and its decision to wait for proposals rather than initiate action indicate that Section 402's primary purpose was to fend off external criticism rather than support internal reevaluation. Furthermore, officials' concern that provider experimentation might become Medicare exploitation made them extremely resistant to proposals for change. Congressional inaction, at least through 1970, reinforced SSA's judgment of the political wisdom of their general approach.

Program Implementation

Both capitation for prepaid group practices and incentive reimbursement were proposals for changes in Medicare reimbursement policy from outside critics. SSA responded to those proposals by doing what they felt was politically necessary without renegotiating the general principles of reimbursement. They took the same approach toward issues that arose within program implementation. SSA's handling of problems in reimbursement between 1966 and 1970 further illustrates its interest in maintaining smooth working relationships with the hospitals without resurrecting the conflicts of 1966.

Once SSA's reimbursement principles were accepted, the agency turned its primary attention to operating the payment program. Although I have not undertaken a review of Medicare's administrative procedures, examples of what they initiated and what they ignored in administration suggest what was important to them. In 1967 BHI took one of its few initiatives in payment policy by introducing Periodic Interim Payments (PIP). According to Thomas Tierney, who became BHI director in 1967, the new proposal would reduce the paperwork necessary to determine interim reimbursement according to hospital bills processed. PIP would instead base interim payments on projected beneficiary utilization and institutional costs, with quarterly adjustments based on actual experience.[86] Despite Tierney's 1967 assessment that the hospitals favored this arrangement,[87] only 800 hospitals actually used PIP through 1972. Apparently most hospitals and intermediaries preferred not to change their standard operating procedures.[88] The proposal itself, however, reflects BHI's concerns in that period. By streamlining the payment process, PIP could reduce inconvenience and delay in hospital payment and therefore ease the working relationship between SSA and the hospitals.

There is a marked contrast between the agency's initiative in this area and its lack of initiative in response to hospitals' manipulation of the reimbursement formula to maximize their Medicare payments. As discussed earlier, the reimbursement formula's allocation methods allowed the hospitals considerable leeway in calculating Medicare's share of their costs. Some of the leeway was inherent in charge-based calculations. Somers and Somers observed: "The word was out early that some hospitals were already redoing their charge structures to take advantage of the RCC formula." They cited one hospital authority who wrote

If Medicare's reimbursement is based on the proportion of a department's charges incurred by old people, it is a simple matter to raise charges selectively in order to raise reimbursement. I heard an administrator say: 'RCC is based on certain hospital statistics but the key statistic is controllable by the hospital.' It is easy and defensible to inflate the prices on services rendered mainly to old people.[89]

The accounting options in Medicare's reimbursement formula reinforced the hospitals' room for maneuver in several ways. First, hospitals were allowed at the start of the program to use the combination method, based on an estimated separation of routine from ancillary service costs. According to a BHI official, these estimates were not monitored by administrators and in fact could be whatever the hospitals chose.[90] Second, the hospitals could choose between the combination method or departmental RCC. Because the combination method lumps all nonroutine service costs together, it pays hospitals more where charge-cost ratios are higher for services the elderly use extensively than for services they use only slightly or not at all. Under these circumstances, the combination method's ratio of beneficiary charges to total charges would be larger than if all charge-cost ratios were the same. The ratio would apply to all hospital service costs, thus subsidizing departments like obstetrics, which have lower ratios.[91]

Since policymakers intentionally made options available to all hospitals, regardless of accounting capability, they were probably not surprised that hospitals were taking advantage of the options.[92] As specific advantages came to their attention, however, BHI considered and explicitly rejected measures to restrict them. According to a later investigation by the General Accounting Office (GAO), intermediaries began to ask questions about the propriety of using the combination method as early as January 1967.[93] One intermediary questioned whether it was appropriate to allow the combination method where it added $528,000 to a hospital's reimbursement. Another asked whether the combination method should be allowed to include such non-Medicare-related costs as delivery rooms.[94] These questions did not go directly to SSA, but to the Blue Cross Association (BCA), which held the primary intermediary contract with SSA. The GAO cited BCA's response:

As a general operating principle, we should not deduct costs from a provider's cost report which the existing rules and regulations allow. As the Medicare Program is refined and changes are introduced, they will be made on a prospective basis so that providers and intermediaries will be able to institute the changes on an equitable basis and with the minimum of friction.[95]

Thus it was up to SSA to direct both the intermediaries and the hospitals in this matter. In late 1967 and 1968 SSA was in fact addressing at least part of this issue. In November 1967, the General Counsel's Office prepared a memorandum for an SSA official on including private room and delivery room costs in reimbursement under the combination method. The first was prohibited by law unless determined medically necessary. The second, the general counsel found, was "clearly in error for the reason that such costs are in no way related to the costs of services furnished to beneficiaries."[96]

Consistent with officials' early commitment to accurate determination of Medicare costs, in May 1968, BHI prepared draft instructions to remedy these problems. The instructions noted cost differences in accommodations; excluded delivery room costs and costs for all services not used by Medicare beneficiaries from allowable costs; and prohibited including charges for those services with total charges in the ratio which determined Medicare's share of costs.[97] SSA never issued these instructions, because of administrative and political concerns. A BHI official described strong internal pressure in the early years of Medicare to maintain the rules with which the program began. It had taken a lot of time and agony, this official recalled, to hammer out a formula and for hospitals and intermediaries to learn to use it. From the administrators' point of view, the program had just begun to work. Bureaucrats responded to proposals for change with "you can't be serious." After all, "we'd have to change all our forms."[98]

Just as change was too much trouble administratively, it appeared to be too much trouble politically. Proposals for payment restrictions were counter to continuing claims for additional payments from 7,000 hospitals and their trade association.[99] SSA accepted these claims, as the standard for payment adequacy without any analysis or investigation of their validity. This suggests the agency's reluctance to disrupt relations with the hospitals, an approach apparent in SSA's defense of existing payment arrangements before congressional committees. BHI Director Tierney explained to the staff of the House Committee on Government Operations that the decision not to implement any new instructions was based on intermediaries' advice to BHI that the new rules would be unfair to the hospitals, because reimbursement did not adequately account for extra nursing costs for the elderly. Furthermore, he explained, the hospitals argued that the cost differential for type of accommodation would create inordinate additional bookkeeping.[100] Senators Ribicoff and Williams of the Finance Committee asked Commissioner Ball about this same issue:

HEW's audit agency has recently criticized your permitting hospitals to elect the combination method of payment, instead of requiring departmental costs. They said this method permits hospitals to pay for private room and delivery costs, both prohibited types of costs under the statute. GAO estimates that the combination method adds some four percent to hospital payments. Do you agree with the HEW audit and GAO?[101]

Commissioner Ball responded that he did not, explaining his position on this issue and on allocation in general in terms of "fairness" to the hospitals.

It seems to me, Senator, the problem we are addressing ourselves to is not how to pay the hospitals of the country the least amount of money. The problem we are addressing ourselves to is how to pay them a fair amount of money for the services they are rendering to the Medicare patient. I can think of other ways you can cut down $100 million or $200 million, but the result might be that people under Blue Cross or the private patient would have to pay them.

What the statute tells us to do is to make sure that we are paying the full cost of the care for the Medicare patient but not for the care of anyone else. . . .

The issue really is, Senator, whether the degree of precision that comes from the departmental method, which the GAO and the HEW audit agency argues ought to be the exclusive method, is now one that is both fair for all institutions and which the great majority of institutions that are using the other method would be able immediately to use.[102]

As BHI Director Tierney explained to the House Committee on Government Operations, if Medicare was paying too much in one area, they were probably paying too little somewhere else.[103]

Thus, five years after SSA first considered and rejected requirements for precise hospital accounting, the agency argued that hospital ability and "fairness" necessitated what Congressman Fountain called a "speculative approach" to reimbursement.[104] Allocation options were initially included in Medicare reimbursement to achieve hospital cooperation; they were apparently retained to maintain it. Asked why the departmental method of apportionment had not been made mandatory, Tierney presented the administrators' dilemma:

You can get accountants who say, well, that is the most accurate accounting method. You are faced, however, in this Nation with 7,000 insitutions whose current and unanimous position is that even under that method and even under the combination method we are not meeting the cost of hospital services to Medicare beneficiaries.

I do not think, Mr. Chairman, that you solve that basic problem by specifying accounting procedures. There have to be some further judgmental factors brought into the picture.[105]

Although Tierney referred to judgments on cost, other policy decisions of that time reveal the greater importance of political judgments. Those decisions related to a major change in SSA's environment, which resulted from the change in administrations in 1969. Medicare, administered as part of a social insurance program by the Social Security Administration, was largely a construct of the Democratic party. Thus, in developing and implementing Medicare, SSA's objectives were consistent with those of the administration in office. Shared ideological goals were reinforced by personal ties, for Medicare was overseen by Wilbur Cohen throughout the sixties. Cohen and chief SSA officials shared experience, goals, and political strategies. As a result, SSA had considerable independence in administering Medicare, with support where necessary from HEW.

The arrival of the Nixon administration in 1969 disrupted this arrangement. Because the administration was new, the president and his secretary of HEW sought to establish control over the numerous agencies of the department, including SSA. This meant that people new to Medicare decision making exercised authority over people who had been with the program and its legislation for a decade. Furthermore, because their political parties were different, the

Republican appointees and the Democratic SSA faced each other with a certain amount of wariness and skepticism. In response to the new administration's approach to hospital reimbursement, SSA elaborated its own political strategy.

When the new president took office, HEW, like other departments, had to review its budget to free some funds for new program initiatives. Both HEW and what was then the Bureau of the Budget (BOB) brought a new perspective to hospital reimbursement. They agreed to eliminate the 2 percent plus factor.[106] A former budget examiner in BOB identified the political and fiscal considerations that made this an "ideal cut": it did not penalize beneficiaries; it eliminated a "windfall" to the providers; and it would save approximately $60 million for each percent. The 2 percent plus factor was a "sop" to get the hospitals to participate in Medicare, said this budget examiner; now that they were in the program, it was no longer necessary.[107]

SSA did not concur in this judgment.[108] They viewed the 2 percent as part of a general agreement they had made with the hospitals, on the basis of which the hospitals went along with Medicare. A senior SSA official found disruption of that agreement "unfair" in two ways: first, it withdrew payment for "unidentified costs" that SSA had accepted as actually incurred; and second, it was a "unilateral decision," made without consultation with the hospitals.[109] In addition to being "unfair," the decision was also unwise, from SSA's perspective. Because the hospitals accepted the 2 percent as reimbursement for expenses they claimed cost far more than that, SSA officials found it a relatively inexpensive way to satisfy the hospitals. Taking it away would resurrect the issues and conflicts of 1966. The 2 percent savings, they believed, was simply not worth the controversy.[110] Furthermore, the department had initiated the controversy without consulting SSA.[111] While this was not the reason for SSA's objections, it no doubt reinforced them.

SSA presented its arguments to HEW officials, but to no avail.[112] The policy went through. The hospitals immediately reacted as the program officials had predicted. A former HEW official recalls that hospitals "descended" on HEW, arguing that the reimbursement formula had not been adequate to start with, particularly with respect to the extra nursing costs for the elderly. In response to this pressure, the undersecretary "backed down" and turned the problem over to SSA with instructions to review reimbursement in consultation with AHA.[113]

If SSA had followed a cost-effectiveness strategy, they might have used this reassessment to increase the accuracy and control of the payment system. Instead, both SSA and the department saw the action and reaction as a validation of SSA's political balance. HEW had tested the political environment and found far greater political pressure for maintaining hospital payment than for restraining it. According to a BHI official, the undersecretary's response was, "Don't let me ever get involved in this again."[114] Thus, he turned reimbursement policy back to the operating agency. The official directive was to identify hospitals' actual costs, pay them, and arrange to pay later for costs incurred but not immediately identifiable.[115] These were not SSA's primary goals, however. Their objective, explained a senior SSA official, was to put at least part of the 2 percent back.[116]

Because of the directive and the Finance Committee's earlier attack on the plus factor as a "bonus" above costs, an SSA official explained, they could not simply reinstitute the 2 percent; rather they looked for a more specific substitute.[117] Officials admitted that the substitute was not "very scientific."[118] SSA took advantage of a pilot study that AHA had undertaken in 1966 when extra nursing costs were central to their claim for greater reimbursement. The study had looked at differentials in nursing costs for patients over and under sixty-five. It found considerable variation. According to an SSA official who consulted on the study, the average figure was useless; what mattered was the situation in each institution. Thus he recommended that the study not be pursued; "no one needed the study to show that all institutions were different."[119]

The inadequacies of the 1966 study did not detract from its convenience as a solution to SSA's problem of restoring reimbursement to earlier levels. Using the study as justification, SSA promulgated regulations that would pay a "nursing differential" of 8.5 percent, that is, 8.5 percent above the hospital's nursing costs for all patients. Estimates of the monetary impact of this differential ranged from one-half to three-quarters of the funds provided by the 2 percent plus.[120]

Substituting the nursing differential for the plus factor was not the only reimbursement change SSA considered in 1969. The substance and politics of those proposals will be reviewed in our discussion of cost control.[121] They do not conflict, however, with the conclusion that SSA approached reimbursement review with a commitment to maintaining its arrangements with the hospitals. That commitment was apparent not only in SSA's goal and method in introducing the nursing differential, but also in the impact of that change on other controversial payment issues. Among SSA's other reasons for not restricting allocation options was the removal of the 2 percent plus. As Commissioner Ball explained to the Senate Finance Committee:

I would not want to argue that over time, it might not be desirable to get to a single method. But I would say that with the other actions that have been taken so far in reducing reimbursement to hospitals, there is great question in my mind whether it would be fair to them at this point to require them all to go to the so-called departmental sophisticated method.[122]

Tierney used a similar argument before the House Government Operations Committee. The contrast between their policy decisions and their claims for reassessment was marked. Tierney agreed with Chairman Fountain that accuracy should be substituted for the "speculative approach" to costs in the existing reimbursement formula. In fact, he said, this was the intent of the review of reimbursement that followed the elimination of the 2 percent plus.[123] At the time he made that claim, however, SSA (supported by HEW) had substituted the nursing differential for the plus factor and rejected internal proposals to revise allocation options. Their approach to decision making was not to investigate and analyze hospital costs, but to maintain arrangements that the hospitals perceived as "fair." The alternative, explained a BHI official, was too complicated to attract the enthusiasm of negotiators and contrary to the operating principle he attributed to the commissioner: the hospitals could ask for more, but the government could not offer less.[124]

Conclusion

When SSA developed its reimbursement principles in 1965-1966, officials were primarily concerned with getting the program under way. Charges that the payment they proposed was inadequate or excessive were withstood on the grounds that the program had to start somewhere, quickly, and that arrangements could be reviewed after the program had operated for a while. But rather than producing reevaluation, experience in operating the Medicare program yielded a commitment to established procedures.

SSA's policy considerations suggest that this commitment did not result from an evenhanded assessment of the costs of change versus its benefits. Officials paid relatively little attention to the potential benefits of change; instead they compared its costs to the comfort of the status quo. Adaptation of the reimbursement formula for GPPPs required administrative changes, would disrupt arrangements with conventional providers and third parties, could antagonize them, and could encourage them to press harder for their demands. It was therefore simpler to have GPPPs conform to the rest of the system.

The calculation on experimentation was similar. Reimbursement experimentation, for the most part, could only be serious if hospitals were required to accept the terms of the experiment. That meant antagonizing hospitals, and neither SSA nor Congress was willing to do that. Freely dispensing funds, on the other hand, might mean increased program costs, potentially antagonizing the Congress as well as conflicting with officials' initial interest in payment efficiency. These were experimentation's political and administrative costs; any benefits were uncertain.

In internal administration, improved working relationships with the hospitals had administrative and political advantages, and initiative therefore occurred. Restricting payment, however, aroused the hospitals' hostility. Again, SSA perceived no benefits that might have countered this cost.

The result of this calculation was to entrench the cost reimbursement principles of 1966, regardless of the consequences in rising costs. As the next chapter shows, this did not mean that SSA had no concern or strategy for cost control; rather their political calculations established the framework within which they pursued cost control. In general, however, administrators found their lives most comfortable if they left well enough alone, and for the most part that was what they did.

Notes

1. Karen Davis, "Hospital Costs and the Medicare Program," *Social Security Bulletin* 36 (August 1973): 19.

2. Ibid., p. 20.

3. Ibid., p. 35.

4. Karen Davis, "Lessons of Medicare and Medicaid for National Health Insurance," Statement Prepared for the Hearings of the Subcommittee on Public Health and Environment, Committee on Interstate and Foreign Commerce, U.S. Congress, December 12, 1973, p. 11. (typewritten), reprinted with permission. Martin Feldstein is generally credited with originating this theory. See Martin S. Feldstein, *The Rising Costs of Hospital Care*, published for the National Center for Health Services Research and Development, U.S. Department of Health, Education, and Welfare (Washington, D.C.: Information Resources Press, 1971).

5. See Davis, "Hospital Costs and the Medicare Program."

6. For a comprehensive review of GPPPs see "The Role of Prepaid Group Practice in Relieving the Medical Care Crisis," Note, *Harvard Law Review* 84 (February 1971): 887-1001.

7. Interview with former official of Group Health Association of America, a trade association for prepaid group practices.

8. Ibid. An interview with a senior SSA official revealed similar ideological commitment to GPPPs. Asked whether he supported GPPPs, he replied, "Of course; that's part of the liberal position."

9. 42 U.S.C. sec. 13951(a)(1). An HEW official, closely involved in Medicare but on the periphery of this particular issue, recalled this language as the result of a "frantic last minute effort in drafting" in response to pressure from the largest GPPP, the Kaiser Health Plan.

10. Excerpts from Report of the Committee on Ways and Means on H.R. 6675, p. 22; and excerpts from Report of the Committee on Finance, U.S. Senate, to Accompany H.R. 6675, p. 24; both in New Members Background Book, Part I, for HIBAC, 1968.

11. This summary is derived from HIBAC Minutes, VIII, April 30-May 1, 1966; XIV, January 7-8, 1967; "Tying Health Insurance Beneficiaries to Group Practice Prepayment Plans," October 1965, discussed in "Experimentation for Prepaying Organizations to Provide Medical Services—Section 402 of the Social Security Act Amendments of 1967," memo from Office of the General Counsel to Mr. Irwin Wolkstein, Division of Policy and Standards, BHI, May 28, 1971,

p. 2, appendix B in "Status of Program Experimentation," Staff Memorandum for HIBAC, November 28, 1972; Howard West, "Group Practice Prepayment Plans in the Medicare Program," *American Journal of Public Health* 59 (April 1969): 624-29; H.F. Newman, "The Impact of Medicare on GPPPs," *American Journal of Public Health* 59 (April 1969): pp. 629-34; H.F. Newman, "Medicare and the Comprehensive Health Cooperative of Puget Sound," *Bulletin of the New York Academy of Medicine* 44 (November 1968): 1321-23; and R.J. Erikson, "The Impact of Medicare on a Group Practice Prepayments Plan," *Bulletin of the New York Academy of Medicine* 44 (November 1968): 1312-20. Although the 1967 HIBAC discussion suggests that physician reimbursement included prospective capitation for in-plan physicians' services, the articles by plan representatives spoke only of retroactively adjusted capitation for physician services.

12. Presentation to HIBAC, XIV:1, January 7, 1967.

13. Minutes, Ibid., pp. 8-9.

14. Ibid., appendix A, November 25, 1966, letter from Glenn Wilson to Lorin Kerr of the Group Health Association of America, following November 22, 1966, meeting between plan representatives and HEW officials, arranged by Wilbur Cohen.

15. Minutes, Ibid., p. 6.

16. See Erikson, "Impact of Medicare," and Newman, "Impact of Medicare."

17. I am indebted to Patrick O'Donoghue, M.D., for clarification of GPPP operations and concerns.

18. For their arguments, see HIBAC Minutes, XIV:1, January 7, 1967.

19. "Report on Response to Problems Posed by Group Practice Prepayment Plans," Staff Report to HIBAC, p. 1, HIBAC Agenda Book, March 4, 1967.

20. Ibid. See also legislative history in Sylvia Law, *Blue Cross: What Went Wrong*, prepared by the Health Law Project, University of Pennsylvania (New Haven: Yale University Press, 1974), pp. 37-38.

21. "Report on Response to Problems Posed by Group Practice Prepayment Plans," pp. 2-3. See also statement to HIBAC of Mel Blumenthal, General Counsel's Office, HIBAC Minutes, XIV:1, January 7, 1967, pp. 20-21.

22. Interview with former BHI official.

23. "Report on Response to Problems Posed by Group Practice Prepayment Plans," p. 3.

24. Statement to HIBAC by Glenn Wilson, Appendix B to HIBAC Minutes, XIV, January 7-8, 1967, pp. 6-7. In his letter to Kerr (see note 14, above), Wilson said:

I believe the time is long overdue for us to insist that Mr. Blumenthal in the office of General Counsel explain this nonsense of conflict of interest. I personally have had this discussion with him at least six times. We keep pointing out the obvious conflict of interest in Blue Cross–Blue Shield and he ignores it. Every time we raise the carrier issue, his only argument is conflict of interest. I urge that we write to Commissioner Ball and insist upon an explanation of how we would be involved in a conflict of interest when Blue Cross–Blue Shield is not so involved.

25. HIBAC Minutes, XIV:1, January 7, 1967, p. 22.

26. Interview.

27. "Report on Response to Problems Posed by Group Practice Prepayment Plans," pp. 4–5. At some point, BHI allowed the plans a capital payment or "equalization factor" in physician reimbursement (Part B), essentially a plus factor intended to equal non-Medicare member payments for noncovered costs. Communication from a GPPP. See Kaiser's request for such a payment, HIBAC minutes, XIV:1, January 7, 1967, p. 14.

28. Interviews with former HEW and BHI officials.

29. Interview with former GHAA official.

30. Interviews reveal that communication between GPPPs and BHI was characterized by hostility and misunderstanding, largely because of their different perspectives.

31. Statement of Dr. George A. Silver, Deputy Assistant Secretary for Health and Scientific Affairs, in U.S., Congress, Senate, Special Committee on Aging, *Cost and Delivery of Health Services to Older Americans, Hearings before the Subcommittee on Health of the Elderly of the Special Committee on Aging*, 90th Cong., 1st sess., June 22–23, 1967, Part I, p. 4.

32. See Wilbur J. Cohen and Robert M. Ball, "Social Security Amendments of 1967: Summary and Legislative History," *Social Security Bulletin* 31 (February 1968): 3–19.

33. The administration convened a National Conference on Medical Care Costs in June 1967; a National Conference on Private Health Insurance in September 1967; a National Conference on Group Practice in October 1967; a National Advisory Commission on Health Facilities; and a Commission on Hospital Effectiveness.

34. As Medicare began, President Johnson requested that the secretary of HEW undertake a study of the reasons for cost increases and the contribution of federal programs to the general inflation. The report, prepared by William Gorham, was submitted to the president in February 1967. "Report to the President on Medical Care Prices," by the Department of Health, Education, and Welfare, in Special Committee on Aging, *Cost and Delivery of Health Services*, appendix 3, pp. 319ff.

35. Senator Anderson introduced a bill on this subject in September 1966. See *Congressional Record*, September 6, 1966, S20884–20888; excerpt included in HIBAC Agenda Book, September 10–11, 1966. The administration introduced a similar amendment in the next session of Congress, "1967 Social Security Recommendations, Summary of Major Proposals," p. 3, HIBAC Agenda Book,

March 4, 1967 and U.S., Congress, House, Committee on Ways and Means, *President's Proposals for Revision in the Social Security System, Hearings before the Committee on Ways and Means on H.R. 5710*, 90th Cong., 1st sess., 1967, pp. 42ff.

36. For testimony on the amendment, see Committee on Ways and Means, *Hearings on H.R. 5710*, pp. 485–486, 700–701, 772–776, 782ff. In the Senate the administration was prepared to make two concessions to get the bill passed: (1) to penalize an institution by not paying it depreciation only upon planning agency *disapproval* of a proposed expenditure; and (2) a positive response to Chairman Long's question whether a planning requirement would be acceptable without a funding requirement. (Interview with participating SSA official and Letter from Secretary Gardner to Senator Long, September 7, 1967, in U.S., Congress, Senate, Committee on Finance, *Social Security Amendments of 1967, Hearings before the Committee on Finance on H.R. 12080*, 90th Cong., 1st sess., p. 725). The committee recommended and the Senate passed legislation in this form, but it was dropped in conference. A participant attributed the amendment's defeat to opposition from the Kaiser Health Plan.

37. See, for example, "Report to the President on Medical Care Prices;" and U.S., President of the United States, "Report of the National Advisory Commission on Health Manpower," November 1967, pp. 55–57.

38. Section 402, H.R. 12080, Social Security Amendments of 1967.

39. See "Reimbursement Under Medicare," *Hospitals J.A.H.A.*, May 16, 1966, appendix D in U.S., Congress, Senate, Committee on Finance, *Reimbursement Guidelines for Medicare*, p. 195; letter from Kermit Gordon, Chairman, HIBAC, to Honorable John W. Gardner, Secretary of HEW, February 9, 1966, appendix C to HIBAC minutes, V, January 28–30, 1966, p. 1; and Committee on Finance, *Reimbursement Guidelines for Medicare*, pp. 108–9.

40. Interview.

41. HIBAC minutes, 1967 and 1968.

42. Interview with former council member.

43. Irwin Wolkstein, "The Legislative History of Hospital Cost Reimbursement," in U.S., Department of Health, Education, and Welfare, Social Security Administration, Office of Research and Statistics, *Reimbursement Incentives for Hospital and Medical Care: Objectives and Alternatives*, Research Report No. 26 (1968), p. 14. Although the publication is dated 1968, the article was written prior to enactment of Section 402. See p. 15.

44. "Incentive Reimbursement Plans Offer a Variety of Approaches to Cost Control," *Hospitals* 43 (June 16, 1969): 63–64.

45. See Katherine G. Bauer and Paul M. Densen, "Some Issues in the Incentive Reimbursement Approach to Cost Containment: An Overview," Health Care Policy Discussion Paper no. 7, May 1973, Harvard Center for Community Health and Medical Care Program on Health Care Policy, Harvard University, Boston, Massachusetts. In this particular case, Bauer and Densen hypothesized

"that the highly favorable local press report of the hospital's accomplishment may have in fact been perceived as the most important reward." Ibid., pp. 38–39, reprinted with permission.

46. "Legislative History Concerning Experiments and Demonstration Projects to Develop Incentives for Economy in the Provision of Health Services," April 1, 1974, provided by BHI, p. 1, dates awareness of the problems of voluntarism at a year or so after enactment. But in early 1968, Senator Long introduced an administration-sponsored amendment authorizing the secretary, on the basis of a successful experiment, to apply the method of reimbursement "to such cases, in such geographical areas, and with respect to such services as he may deem appropriate"—including those beyond the scope of the experiment. (S. 3323 to amend Section 402 of the Social Security Amendments of 1967; reported in SSA's "Commissioner's Bulletin" of April 19, 1968, no. 73, p. 2, included in HIBAC Agenda Book, April 27-28, 1968.) This amendment was never acted upon and may have been simply a public relations measure, intended to suggest activity. On the other hand, since it would allow the secretary to impose a reimbursement method, it may have been a way of dealing with the problem of voluntarism.

47. "Legislative History Concerning Experiments," p. 2.

48. Interview.

49. Interview with SSA legislative official.

50. Interview with BHI officials.

51. Interview with BHI official.

52. "Status of Program Experimentation in the Bureau of Health Insurance," Staff Memorandum for HIBAC, November 28, 1972.

53. Ibid., p. 6.

54. Ibid., pp. 6-7.

55. Interview with BHI official.

56. HIBAC, "Status of Program Experimentation," November 28, 1972, p. 1.

57. Ibid., pp. 6-7.

58. "Incentive Reimbursement Experimentation Program," Staff Memorandum for HIBAC, p. 2, in HIBAC Agenda Book, November 16-17, 1968.

59. HIBAC, "Status of Program Experimentation," November 28, 1972, pp. 7-8.

60. Ibid., p. 7.

61. "Incentive Reimbursement Experimentation Program," Staff Report for HIBAC, HIBAC Agenda Book, April 27-28, 1968, p. 2 and attachment A, Guideline 7.

62. BHI, "Legislative History Concerning Experiments," p. 1.

63. HIBAC, "Incentive Reimbursement Experimentation Program," April 27-28, 1968, p. 8. Experiment proposed by the Associated Hospital Service of New York.

64. Ibid., p. 8.

65. Interview with BHI official. Eight of the original eighteen participants withdrew, including the largest ones. Communication from BHI.

66. Ibid., and HIBAC, "Status of Program Experimentation," November 28, 1972, p. 8.

67. See "Report to the President on Medical Care Prices," appendix 3 to Special Committee on Aging, *Costs and Delivery of Services to Older Americans*, pp. 319ff.

68. Summary notes by Robert M. Cunningham, Jr., editor, *Modern Hospital*, in "Report to the President," *Costs and Delivery of Services,* pp. 167ff.

69. Excerpts from Report of the Committee on Ways and Means on H.R. 12080, p. 43, and excerpts from Report of the Committee on Finance, U.S. Senate, on H.R. 12080, p. 71; both in New Members Background Book, Part I, for HIBAC, 1968.

70. HIBAC, "Incentive Reimbursement Experimentation Program," April 27-28, 1968, p. 2 and Attachment D, p. 2.

71. Guideline 1(c), Guidelines for Incentive Reimbursement Experiments, Attachment A, to HIBAC, "Incentive Reimbursement Experimentation Program," April 27-28, 1968.

72. "Incentive Reimbursement and Group Practice Prepayment," presented at 19th Annual Group Health Institute, New York City, May 4-6, 1969, *Proceedings*, p. 92.

73. That is, if capitation were equal to Medicare nonmember beneficiary costs in the same area. See Mildred Corbin and Aaron Krute, "Some Aspects of Medicare Experience with Group Practice Prepayment Plans," *Social Security Bulletin* 38 (March 1975): 3-11. Although the authors emphasize that the plans studied cannot be considered representative of plans participating in Medicare, five of the seven had lower reimbursement levels for their beneficiary members than for beneficiary nonmembers in the same area.

74. 19th Annual Group Health Institute, *Proceedings*, pp. 98-99.

75. Interview with former GHAA official.

76. The experiment (with New York's HIP) was originally described as intended "to test a single capitation payment . . ." HIBAC, "Status of Program Experimentation," November 1968, p. 2. In the 1972 review of the experiment for HIBAC, capitation was not mentioned, and in interviews it was explained that capitation reimbursement was not what was being investigated. Rather, a BHI official explained, it was a test of medical care management under a GPPP. Capitation was the basis for comparing costs inside and outside the experiment, with HIP receiving a share of any difference where its costs were lower, but overall reimbursement continued to be on the previously established basis. Since Medicare would previously have paid for hospital use that HIP was able to eliminate, the program saved the difference between the cost and the reward payment to HIP. This experiment was regarded by a generally skeptical SSA official as quite useful. For a report on the experiment, see Ellen W. Jones,

Paul M. Densen, Isidore Altman, Sam Shapiro, and Howard West, "HIP Incentive Reimbursement Experiment: Utilization and Costs of Medical Care 1969 and 1970," *Social Security Bulletin* 37 (December 1974): 3–34.

77. See above. p. 91.

78. For HIBAC attitudes on capitation and GPPPs, see U.S., Department of Health, Education, and Welfare, Social Security Administration, Bureau of Health Insurance, *Health Insurance Benefits Advisory Council Annual Report on Medicare, Covering the Period July 1, 1966 to December 31, 1967* (Washington, D.C.: July 1969), pp. 31 and 38; and HIBAC Minutes, XXX, January 10, 1970, pp. 7, 9 and appendix A, letter from Chairman Charles Schultze to Secretary of HEW Robert Finch.

79. Interview with BHI official.

80. Bert Seidman, AFL–CIO, in U.S., Congress, Senate, Committee on Government Operations, *Health Care in America: Hearings before the Subcommittee on Executive Reorganization of the Committee on Government Operations*, 90th Cong., 2d sess., April 1968, pp. 742–43.

81. Ibid., p. 509.

82. Ibid., pp. 513 and 520–521. See also material submitted to the committee by Dr. Lee, including the National Advisory Committee on Health Manpower's report on Kaiser and the planning history of the Cleveland Community Health Foundation. Lee commented that while the data did not permit firm conclusions, there was increasing data that demonstrated that quality and cost controls could be achieved in prepaid group practice and neighborhood health centers.

83. Bauer and Densen, p. 59, reprinted with permission.

84. Ibid., p. 59.

85. Ibid., p. 60.

86. HIBAC minutes, clearance draft, XVII, September 16, 1967, pp. 6–7.

87. Ibid.

88. Interview with BHI official.

89. Steven Sieverts, Associate Executive Director, Hospital Planning Association of Allegheny County, Letter to Arthur Hess, Director, Bureau of Health Insurance, May 5, 1966. Quoted in Herman M. Somers and Anne R. Somers, *Medicare and the Hospitals* (Washington, D.C.: The Brookings Institution, 1967), pp. 168–69.

90. Interview.

91. I am indebted to Karen Davis for clarifying this issue.

92. For HIBAC concerns, see HIBAC Minutes, IV:1, January 7, 1966, pp. 10–12. Hospital accountants also spoke of manipulation in testimony before the Ways and Means Committee on H.R. 5710 in 1967. The Southwestern Pennsylvania Chapter of the American Association of Hospital Accountants challenged SSA's justification for step-down cost finding as an improvement in accounting, and for RCC as a fair division of costs among various patient groups.

They considered both assumptions erroneous because cost finding was used in making management decisions, while reimbursement reports were intended to maximize reimbursement. Thus cost finding for Medicare was not directed at better management but at getting the most money. Consequently, it discouraged better management and better cost control through accounting. The argument seems to be that any accounting required by Medicare would be distorted, and therefore should not be required. U.S., Congress, House, Committee on Ways and Means, *President's Proposals for Revision of the Social Security System: Hearings on H.R. 5710*, 90th Cong., 1st sess., 1967, p. 2252.

93. U.S., General Accounting Office, *Lengthy Delays in Settling the Costs of Health Services Furnished Under Medicare*, Social Security Administration, Department of Health, Education, and Welfare, Report to the Congress by the Comptroller General of the United States, June 23, 1971, p. 23.

94. Ibid., p. 23.

95. Ibid., p. 23.

96. Ibid., p. 24.

97. Ibid., p. 29.

98. Interview with BHI official. Operational problems with change are also apparent from Tierney's explanation to the Senate Finance Committee of decisions to retain fiscal agents that were performing poorly:

The basic problem, I am sure you can understand, is that no matter how poor a carrier may have been in the beginning, they now have spent maybe four years developing personnel, computer capacity, technique, and in improving their abilities. It becomes a very difficult judgmental question—shall you throw that full four years out of the window and start all over with the new carrier, even though the new carrier may have demonstrated a good capacity in another area, can it now come in and take over this area? [U.S., Congress, Senate, Committee on Finance, *Medicare and Medicaid: Hearings,* 91st Cong., 2d sess., 1970, p. 134.]

Similarly, before the House Government Operations Committee, Tierney explained:

We would have to find a new intermediary and the new intermediary would have to establish new relationships with the hospitals, they would have to establish their own process, they would have to have their own personnel and find their own space, and hopefully, because of a past record of better performance elsewhere, you come out with a better performance. But it's an extremely painful transition.

Our hope to date has been that we could improve the performance of this intermediary and bring down its cost and get it on an acceptable level. If we become convinced that we can't, we will make the change but where we make the change, things are going to be pretty rough for awhile. . . .

This is one of the limitations that concerns us, frankly. This is our ultimate weapon, to terminate a contract, and it is a kind of overkill in many ways. [U.S., Congress, House, Committee on Government Operations, Hearings before the

Subcommittee of the Committee on Government Operations, 91st Cong., *Administration of Federal Health Benefits Program*, 1st sess., February and March 1970, Part I, p. 203.]

99. See, for example, AHA testimony, Committee on Ways and Means, *Hearings on H.R. 5710*, pp. 691ff.

100. Committee on Government Operations, *Administration of Federal Health Benefit Programs*, pp. 79–80.

101. Committee on Finance, *Medicare and Medicaid: Hearings*, 1970; Senator Ribicoff, p. 73; Senator Williams, p. 121.

102. Ibid., p. 74. Similar statement by Tierney, pp. 121–22.

103. Committee on Government Operations, *Administration of Federal Health Benefit Programs*, pp. 32ff., especially pp. 34–39, and 44–48.

104. Ibid., p. 48.

105. Ibid., p. 47.

106. Within the department, officials attributed the decision to undersecretary John Veneman, according to interviews.

107. Interview.

108. Interviews with HEW, SSA, and BHI officials.

109. Interview with senior SSA official.

110. Interviews with SSA and BHI officials.

111. Interviews with HEW, SSA, and BHI officials.

112. Interviews with SSA and BHI officials.

113. Interview with HEW official.

114. Interview with BHI official.

115. A BHI official attributed this direction to the undersecretary.

116. Interview with senior SSA official.

117. Ibid.

118. Ibid.

119. Interview with official in SSA's Office of Research and Statistics. Criticism has also been leveled at the study's methodology, including the charge that the personnel who conducted the study knew its objective. For a general critique, see Law, *Blue Cross*, pp. 86–88.

120. Interviews with HEW and SSA officials. Robert J. Myers, former SSA chief actuary, estimated it as half. See Robert J. Myers, *Medicare*, published for McCahon Foundation, Bryn Mawr, Pennsylvania (Homewood, Ill.: Richard D. Irwin, 1970), p. 134.

121. See chapter 6.

122. Committee on Finance, *Medicare and Medicaid: Hearings*, 1970, p. 74. Similar statement by Tierney, pp. 121–22.

123. Committee on Government Operations, *Administration of Federal Health Benefit Programs*, pp. 42–43, 45, and 48.

124. Interview.

**Containing Hospital Costs:
Political Peace and Bureaucratic
Control**

With Medicare, Medicaid, and private insurance providing a steady flow of funds
to the medical industry, hospital and physician costs rose rapidly in the 1960s
and 1970s, continually outpacing inflation in the rest of the economy.[1] Hospital
costs per day more than doubled between 1966 and 1972.[2] Contributing to and
reflecting these increases, Medicare hospital insurance expenditures have continually exceeded estimates and scheduled payroll tax revenues.[3] By 1969, costs
as a percentage of payroll were double what had been predicted in 1965, and
actuaries estimated the deficit in the trust fund over the next twenty-five years
at $126 billion. In February 1970, SSA's Chief Actuary Robert Myers reesti-
mated the deficit at $216 billion. Congress increased the taxable wage base and
tax rates to cover these deficits and additional benefits, beginning in 1967 and
continuing into the early 1970s. By 1973 Congress had raised the taxable wage
base from $6,600 to $10,800 (with additional increases scheduled through
1974, rising thereafter with the rise in wages), and had promulgated an actual
tax rate over 60 percent higher than 1965 predictions.

Although the tax that finances Medicare remains relatively low,[4] cost increases have had significant impact. Under the law, beneficiaries are responsible
for a share of hospital costs—specifically, an initial payment or deductible equal
to the average cost for a day in the hospital and a percentage of that average for
each day in the hospital after an initial sixty days.[5] In 1966, the deductible was
$40; in 1970, $52; in 1972, $68. At this writing (summer, 1976), it is over $100.[6]

Compounded by increasing use of services in Medicare and rising enrollment
in Medicaid, rising costs have also had a major impact on the federal budget. In
1967, Medicare and Medicaid cost the federal government $4.5 and $1.2 billion
respectively and represented 66 percent of budget obligations for health programs.[7] In fiscal 1974, they cost $11.3 and $5.8 billion. Their combined total
is expected to be $25 billion in fiscal 1976 and $30.4 billion in fiscal 1977.
That last increase, $5.4 billion, is equivalent to the administration's total budget
request for all other health programs for that year.[8]

Because the expenditures of Medicare and Medicaid are mandated in the
law and are not subject to annual appropriations, they are frequently characterized as "uncontrollable" budget expenses. Charles Schultze explained the effect
of the "uncontrollables" on other program expenditures in the late 1960s.

Since it seemed unconscionable to cut back on payments going directly to the
neediest Americans—the freeze on welfare payments voted by the Congress

111

was never put into effect—strenuous efforts were made to hold the line or to cut back on other programs to offset the fiscal effects of the "uncontrollables"....

In 1968 and 1969, the growth of education and health programs (except Medicare and Medicaid) virtually ceased, despite rising costs. Construction of hospitals and college buildings was delayed and several shifts were made from grant to loan financing to get programs "off the budget."[9]

John Iglehart described the same situation in 1976:

The increase in health costs will be a major factor in shaping the Ford Administration's entire domestic policy agenda in election year 1976.

"The health cost increases will put a squeeze on every other program budget in town," a ranking HEW official predicted.[10]

One of the programs affected by the rising costs of medical care and existing federal health insurance has been a national health insurance program to cover those people who still lack public or private insurance protection.[11] Despite extensive consideration of legislation to resolve this problem, no action has been taken. Reluctance to increase the government's financial burden—particularly at a time of general concern about federal spending—and to take on responsibility for medical cost inflation and its control have contributed significantly to this result.[12]

This history suggests that inflation in medical costs has affected other government programs more than Medicare. As Schultze recognized,[13] however, what is called "uncontrollable" is not immune to control. Whether and how to control Medicare expenditures are choices that have confronted Medicare policymakers since 1965. Theoretically, these choices include explicit reduction or elimination of the benefits Medicare originally offered. Our focus, however, will be on controlling payments while maintaining benefits, that is, controlling expenditures to hospitals. How Medicare officials viewed their responsibility for such control would have varied with their political strategy. If they had pursued a cost-effectiveness strategy, policymakers might have initiated payment changes to control costs, either by restricting reimbursement or by improving the market for hospital services. A balancing strategy would have led SSA to control costs in response to officials' perceptions of political pressure.

In fact, consistent with their initial stance on hospital reimbursement, SSA officials had an agenda for cost containment—specifically, to restrict and avoid reimbursement they considered excessive. At the same time, however, they did not wish to disrupt their working relationship with the hospitals. As a result, SSA pursued cost containment in response to outside political pressure. Evidence of SSA's agenda and its strategy comes from officials' assessment of the cost problem and possible solutions; the timing and scope of the solutions actually pursued; and SSA's reactions to cost control measures initiated by others.

After 1968, SSA's judgments were not necessarily government policy on Medicare, nor was Medicare policy the only government policy that affected medical cost containment. Although we will discuss other factors and policies, this is not a comprehensive account of federal policy on medical costs. Rather, it illustrates how officials charged with program operations perceived their responsibilities and interests in a political environment.

Agenda and Actions When Pressure Was Low

In January 1970, BHI officials prepared materials for HIBAC that revealed their perception of the cost problem and appropriate solutions.[14] First, they explained to HIBAC the kinds of choices cost control entailed.

As we believe these papers demonstrate, there seem to be no magic bullets that will control medical costs without direct or indirect restriction on physicians and providers, control program costs in face of rising medical costs without disadvantage to the beneficiary, or insulate the beneficiary from rising medical and program costs without increased cost to the general taxpayer or the social security contributor. What must be faced in evaluating the Administration's present policy is the hard trade-off of interest involved in adopting alternative policies. The Council may wish to give its advice on the value judgments underlying such tradeoffs. The major interests involved in the delivery and financing of medical care are represented on the Council and trade-offs acceptable to the Council may be acceptable to the Nation as a whole.[15]

An official recalled that he did not intend this memorandum to evoke council action. On the contrary, reflecting his skeptical view of the council, he sought to avoid "glib" discussion of the issues. He characterized his message: "If you're serious about cost control, think about these."[16]

After elaborating the multitude of technical, political, and philosophical issues that cost containment entailed, the memorandum addressed Medicare's contribution to medical cost inflation and what might be done about it:

It appears likely that there is a circular situation in connection with hospital costs and what is paid for care. The more that costs rise, the more hospitals demand for payment. The more that people pay for care (the more income hospitals have), the more that hospitals will spend (have as costs). Most hospitals do not pay dividends or support housing for the poor when they have extra funds. They use almost all available funds to build up their own services. An increment that, in the first instance, permits the financing of an increase in services may produce a permanent increase in operating costs, not only for depreciation on any capital investment involved but for the staff and supplies used in operating the new service.

Medicare is in theory a cost reimbursement system, so that it might be said that no increment to hospital services is financed by Medicare. However, it is not entirely correct that Medicare payments to hospitals provide no profit. In the case of physicians' services where the physician is on a salary, but his services are paid for on a fee-for-service basis, a profit is normally generated by the hospital. Furthermore, if Medicare pays full cost for regular services, the hospital generates a profit on extras paid for by Medicare patients. Finally, Medicare leaves open a number of options (most prominent being a choice of departmental or combination method) on cost calculation among which the hospital may choose the most favorable. Any cost reimbursement methods is only approximate and the choice of the most favorable options may generate a profit. Profits such as these may tend to support increases in services and costs. In addition, the presence of assured income, and the reduction in unpaid services that accompanied Medicare and Medicaid, facilitate the expansion of services in part by making borrowing easier.

While increases in services are often desirable, it must be recognized that one avenue for cost control is simply to tighten up on reimbursement. One question, then, is how reimbursement can be tightened up within the reasonable cost concept. One method would be to eliminate some or all the options now available in computing costs. Another method, consistent with the Medicare approach to the prevailing charge limit in establishing reasonable charges, would be to rule as nonreimbursable costs found to be substantially out of line with costs of comparable institutions. New York State has, in effect, taken such a step in establishing that institutions whose routine costs are more than 10 percent above the average for their group will not be reimbursed above the ceiling by Blue Cross or Medicaid. Similarly, maximums might be set on durations of stay reimbursable for various treatments. It could be established that a hospital that had average stays for a given treatment that exceeded a designated ceiling would not be reimbursed for care beyond the maximum covered.[17]

As an alternative to adjusting cost reimbursement, the memorandum suggested policies that would require or induce changes in the medical delivery system. Among these were rate setting (along public utility lines) and community planning. The memorandum questioned the first as complex and the second as inadequate to resolve or overrule the "often sharp conflicts between community advantage and individual institution advantage."[18]

The question arises as to how the conflict between the interests of the community and those of individual units of the health system may be reduced. One way would be to increase the size of the unit under a single management. For example, if all hospitals in a community were under a single management, many of the present planning difficulties would probably be minimal. The management plan of a unit owning all of a community's health facilities would be much more nearly equivalent to a community plan. The advantages that largeness in scale have given to other aspects of American enterprise would tend to apply to health as well. The further question might be, how can the system of medical care be transformed into this new shape. Control of new capital, a critical item, has been proposed as an answer.

Some ways that have been proposed to add controls to capital input are:

(1) Cease making depreciation payments as part of reimbursement.

(2) Make all depreciation payments and other capital payments to a pooled community fund to be dispensed only to the advantage of system improvement.

(3) Modify the rules for providing capital funds to provide that grants would be conditioned on their effect on the efficiency of the system. They could be granted where the use would directly lower cost. If they were to be granted to provide an additional service, then priority could be given to organizations that demonstrate a capacity to handle the funds efficiently and that would pass through efficiency gains to the consumer. Furthermore, priority for grants for new services could be given to existing organizations to increase scale rather than to new small units. Finally, grants might be denied to an organization that requests funds for one project, but intends to use other funds for other low priority purposes or has funds available that might be used for such other purposes.

However, dependence on a grant authority to direct the change in health systems requires a very wise authority, and such wisdom is hard to come by. Further, if such an authority is to be successful, it must have the power to overcome the difficulties of the Hill-Burton and other programs that have often acted in favor of local interests, sometimes to the disadvantage of the health system. The end effect of statutory or regulatory authority control to improve the efficiency of the health system depends, in the case of power over capital as in any other control, on whether, and if so how, the power is used.[19]

In sum, the memorandum identified open-ended Medicare reimbursement as a major contribution to hospital cost inflation and proposed restrictions on payment as a solution. One way to control hospital spending was simply to pay them less. We have already seen evidence of BHI's interest in controlling payment excesses in officials' initial recommendations on hospital reimbursement in 1965, their refusal to open reimbursement under the experimental authority of Section 402, and proposed changes in allocation during 1967 and 1968. Although some of the most drastic measures posed in the memorandum were never seriously considered, BHI officials did try to establish limits on hospital reimbursement from 1969 on. However, in the absence of political pressure for government control, SSA's actions fell significantly short of officials' objectives.

As officials themselves acknowledged to HIBAC, SSA had made no effort before 1969 to define "reasonable" cost reimbursement.[20] Limits on individual hospital reimbursement were discussed in congressional hearings before Medicare's enactment. The emphasis then was on SSA's general intention to pay each hospital the cost it incurred, as provided in the AHA principles. But officials acknowledged and Congress explicitly recognized an exception to that rule,[21] also included in the AHA principles,

where a particular institution's costs are found to be substantially out of line with those of institutions similar in size, scope of services, utilization and other relevant factors.[22]

In the 1969 reassessment of reimbursement that followed the elimination of the 2 percent plus, officials proposed to use this authority in a limited form. BHI informed HIBAC that in an effort to "intensify scrutiny" of reasonableness of costs, they planned to require institutions whose costs were out of line with those of other institutions to justify their costs. A first step in this policy was a letter to intermediaries, instructing them to restrict payments for specific hospital costs to the cost a "prudent buyer" would pay.[23]

As it turned out, the "prudent buyer" instructions were also the last step in this effort. BHI officials recalled attempting to define reasonable cost ceilings for extended care facilities (ECFs), specifically, at the level of hospital costs. In their view, this ceiling was easily defensible since Medicare had included ECFs *because* they were less expensive than hospitals. Nevertheless, they reported, HEW's general counsel found the ceiling beyond SSA's legal authority. These officials disagreed but did not press further. As a former official explained, bureaucrats had to decide where to direct their energy. They could initiate or "send up" an unpopular proposal, but pushing it seemed a waste of time.[24]

In contrast to the general restrictions these officials proposed, the January 1970 memorandum characterized measures SSA had actually taken as "piecemeal" solutions to "problem cases."[25] With few exceptions, these measures focused on exploitation of federal payment for personal gain. Thus, SSA limited reimbursement for purchases from related organizations, payments to institutional owners, reimbursement of franchise fees to the value of management services, and reimbursement of advertising costs to the value of information services.[26] Similarly, the prudent buyer policy simply encouraged using the market price as a "reasonable" standard for hospital purchases. The few measures likely to have greater impact on hospital practices encountered obstacles. A limit on Medicare's share of empty bed costs, for example, required a definition of adequate staff levels, which was causing some difficulty, and adjustment of a 1966 concession, accelerated depreciation, was still in the planning stages months after officials had identified abuse.[27]

Comparing the actions SSA considered with those they took shows how they restricted their initiatives to the legally and politically safest sphere—responding to fraud or near-fraud. Despite officials' awareness of a far broader problem, SSA was unwilling to take the more controversial step of restricting their open-ended reimbursement to each institution for the costs it incurred.

A similar contrast between perception and action appears in legislative proposals at this time. In July 1969, President Nixon took a dramatic stance on health policy. Introducing a new assistant secretary for Health and a report on the health care system, he told a press conference:

We face a massive crisis in this area and unless action is taken, both administratively and legislatively, to meet this crisis within the next two or three years, we will have a breakdown in our medical care system which could have consequences affecting millions of people throughout this country.[28]

The crisis was the "crippling inflation" of medical costs. Among their proposals to deal with this and other problems, the administration announced consideration of a number of cost control amendments for Medicare. Except for reintroducing a tie between capital reimbursement and planning, the administration's amendments introduced no major changes in reimbursement practices. According to a participating official, the administration spent the next year and a half searching for a response to the "crisis" they had announced. The legislative proposals of 1969, he said, showed how they were "stretching to find something to do."[29] As elaborated in the summer and fall of 1969, the administration proposed the following: discontinuing reimbursement for services of certain suppliers of services on evidence of gross abuse; payment of hospital charges where charges were less than costs; withholding reimbursement for depreciation and interest expenses where they were attributable to capital expenditure which a state planning agency had determined as not conforming to its overall plan; including noncovered services and requiring institutional participation in reimbursement experiments; requiring, as a condition of institutional participation, a corporate plan with operating and capital expenditures budgets; determining the "medical necessity" of hospital admissions as well as long stays; and expanding authority to deal with overpayments to institutions.[30] As Commissioner Robert Ball explained to the Ways and Means Committee:

These are important changes but no one would for a minute suggest that they will reverse the trend of rising medical prices, which is related to long-range factors of supply and demand and to increasing costs in the operation of hospitals. But I do believe that these changes would improve our ability to hold down the increase.[31]

In contrast to the BHI memorandum for HIBAC, there was no hint here of Medicare's contribution to this "trend." On the contrary, Ball's statement implied that its causes were outside the scope of the program, and he was not publicly challenged at that time.

Responses to Pressure

When Medicare policy *was* publicly challenged, SSA and HEW responded with more aggressive policy positions. Their most dramatic policy proposal was largely rhetorical and had little substance behind it. But congressional criticism created an environment in which BHI officials were able to undertake at least three measures they had earlier advocated unsuccessfully. That SSA waited for political consensus before initiating changes is evidence of its balancing strategy. The changes actually made are evidence of SSA's agenda for cost containment.

In 1969 the Senate Finance Committee staff undertook an investigation of Medicare administration. In their preliminary report in July, the staff argued that the administration of Medicare is inadequate and ineffective from the standpoint of insistence upon proper cost controls and utilization review. There is a high degree of tolerance for carriers and intermediaries who cannot reasonably be considered as "efficient and economical" as required by law. There is a lack of current program information with respect to costs and utilization which hampers both effective administration and estimating.

In their eagerness to get as much health care as possible to the greatest number of people, secondary concern seems to have been given to the quality of the care and the control of the costs. The resulting severe actuarial deficiencies which have occurred in Medicare are then glossed over with statements that congress need merely increase the Social Security tax, or wage base and the costs can be paid.[32]

Like BHI officials, the Finance Committee staff perceived uncontrolled payments to hospitals as a major contribution to inflation and proposed solutions ranging from elimination of fraud to ceilings on reimbursement increases. Finance Committee staff and BHI personnel had worked together closely since before Medicare began. As a result of the two staffs' frequent communication, similar perspectives, and shared data, their evaluations were markedly similar.[33]

In July 1969 and February 1970, the Finance Committee staff criticized Medicare cost reimbursement generally for its encouragement of inefficiency and inflation and specifically for such elements as its "blanket" award of plus factors—whether the 2 percent or the nursing differential; its "disproportionate" share of empty bed costs; and its invitation to manipulate depreciation allowances.[34] The February hearings also included an attack on the persistence of allocation options.[35] Along with specific remedies where appropriate, the staff called the committee's attention to the provisions of proposed legislation (S. 1195) "designed to provide a basis for moderate and reasonable controls on payments to hospitals and extended care facilities under medicare and medicaid."[36] Provisions included payment of an institutions charges where less than costs; limiting Medicare's recognition of a hospital's annual increase in operating (noncapital) costs to the annual percentage increase in the Medical Care Price Index for that geographic or metropolitan area; and denial of capital reimbursement where a planning agency disapproved a major capital investment. In addition the staff proposed that the committee consider

limiting reimbursement for care provided in a given institution to not more than a reasonable difference above the costs for comparable care and services in a similar institution in the same area.[37]

The staff also criticized as inadequate both intermediaries' handling of reimbursement and SSA's supervision of intermediaries. Citing conflicts of interest, the staff recommended that intermediaries be designated by HEW rather than nominated by the hospitals.[38] BHI officials had made a similar suggestion to HIBAC in May 1969.[39]

None of the problems or solutions the Finance Committee staff identified was new to SSA, but by altering SSA's perceptions of the relative costs and benefits of change versus the status quo, this public critique increased the agency's inclination to act—both by reducing SSA's comfort with existing practices and by reducing the resistance they perceived from the hospitals. The Finance Committee staff report and hearings made senior SSA officials decidedly uncomfortable. One described the hearings as "deliberately unbalanced, unfair, sensationalized and wrong."[40] Anticipating this, officials tried to "turn things around," both by taking the offensive with some positive recommendations, and by focusing on the Medicare law rather than administration as the source of the problem.[41] Accordingly, recalled an official involved in legislation, agency staff hurried to develop proposals for the February hearings. Compared to the legislative amendments discussed above, he said, the new proposals were "real blockbusters."[42] The administration proposed to replace the entire system of retrospective hospital cost reimbursement with prospectively set payments, and to limit reimbursable fee increases for physicians to a price index.[43]

Prospective reimbursement was an expansion of the incentive reimbursement concept with which SSA had supposedly been experimenting. Its basic premise was that letting hospitals know their revenues before rather than after they incurred expenses would enhance their fiscal responsibility. By 1970, this premise had become conventional wisdom on hospital payment, adopted by health experts and the health industry[44] as well as the government. Irwin Wolkstein of BHI contrasted the interests of the payers and hospitals in the new approach:

AHA's interest in the prospective approach seems to arise from a desire for a firm commitment from the contracting agencies before a contemplated expenditure is made, that each of the agencies will pay its share of the expenditure. . . .

Contracting agencies, on the other hand, have been attracted to certain forms of prospective reimbursement as substitutes for retroactive reasonable cost reimbursement since denial of expenses after the fact because they are unreasonable had proved generally impractical.[45]

Thus, although both parties could agree on payment in advance, they still could not agree on what payment should include or how high it should be. A BHI official emphasized that prospective reimbursement was a mechanism, not a policy. As their handling of incentive reimbursement experiments had revealed, when it came to policy BHI officials were extremely skeptical of "rewards" for efficiency. Rewards, they believed, would only be spent. To them, the only effective way to contain costs was to contain or limit reimbursement.[46] Neither this policy question nor any other was addressed in the legislative proposal of February 1970. As a legislative official summed it up, "the testimony was it."[47] A BHI official recalled the commissioner's comments: "We've announced it.

Now figure out what we meant."[48] Consistent with a balancing strategy, SSA committed itself as far as consensus existed and no further.

SSA's and HEW's response was partially successful in "stealing headlines," but it produced other results whose impact was perhaps more lasting. Although senior SSA officials were embarrassed by public criticism, they acknowledged their willingness to use it. Before the Finance Committee hearings, one official reported, the only pressure in Medicare administration was from hospitals, physicians, and others for less government control. With the powerful Senate Finance Committee advocating more control, he said, SSA could exercise greater authority.[49]

Legislative Action

A major exercise of authority followed from congressional reactions to the prospective reimbursement proposal. The proposal first received legislative consideration in executive sessions of the Ways and Means Committee at the end of February 1970. Although the administration proposed that they be granted authority to implement prospective reimbursement as they saw fit, a participating SSA official reported that the committee immediately reduced the proposal to an experimental level.[50] The House and Senate ultimately enacted an amendment directing the secretary to develop large-scale experiments and demonstration projects to test various methods of prospective reimbursement. The amendment required detailed reports to the Ways and Means and Finance Committees on the results of experimentation. Authority to implement a new approach to reimbursement without further congressional consideration was not granted. Moreover, despite their acknowledgement of HEW's argument that mandatory hospital participation was necessary to achieve broad coverage, Congress did not give HEW authority to require hospitals to participate in experiments.[51]

The committee was no more convinced that prospective reimbursement in and of itself would solve cost problems than were BHI staff. After outlining the purported advantage of prospective reimbursement—encouraging efficiency through the prospect of gain and the risk of loss—the committee identified potential disadvantages in its report:

While it is clear, for example, that prospective rate setting will provide incentives for health care institutions to keep costs at a level no higher than the rates set, it is not clear that the rates set would result in government reimbursement at levels lower than, or even as low as, that which would result under the present retroactive cost finding approach. Providers could be expected to press for a rate that would cover all the costs, including research costs and bad debts, as well as margins of safety in the prospective rates that might result in reimbursement—if their requests were met—in excess of the costs that would have been reimbursed under the present approach. Moreover, any excess of reimbursement over costs to voluntary providers would probably be used to expand services, and the new level of expenditures might be reflected in setting higher prospective rates for future years.[52]

An additional amendment, generated by Ways and Means staff in discussion with BHI, further revealed the committee's skepticism. In the words of one BHI official, the amendment was a one-way grant of authority to implement prospective reimbursement—setting limits, not providing rewards.[53] BHI had unsuccessfully pursued this objective administratively some months before; now, in conjunction with committee staff, they obtained legislative backing for the introduction of "reasonable" limits on individual hospital costs. What had previously been expressed only in committee reports—the denial of costs out of line with those of similar institutions—would now be included in the statute itself. The action further strengthened their hand, BHI officials believed, by authorizing the establishment of limits in advance, eliminating the political and technical difficulties of denying costs already incurred.

A basic problem in acting after the fact against an institution that has had excessive costs by paying less than the cost experienced is that someone must cover the deficiency. The only way out of this dilemma is to attempt to identify potential excessive costs before they occur and to prevent this occurrence.[54]

The legislative history of this amendment verifies administrators' perceptions of limited support for regulatory action. Although the proposal's initial objective was to discourage inefficiency, legislative discussion turned instead to eliminating "luxury." The Ways and Means Committee specified that limits should be set sufficiently above the average cost per patient day so that only cases with extraordinary expenses would be subject to limits.[55] The Senate Finance Committee, who had been so critical of SSA's failure to control costs, proposed that a test of "gross" inefficiency rather than simple inefficiency be the basis for cost limits.[56] This provision was dropped in the House-Senate conference.

Despite these qualifications, BHI officials perceived the measure as a first step in cost control activity. They were skeptical of more detailed control activities, like planning and budgeting. When he was BHI Deputy Director of Policy Planning, Irwin Wolkstein discussed publicly the technical and political problems of budget review:

This example presupposes that the know-how will exist to determine whether inefficiency exists—whether, for example, administrative costs are too high—or quality of services—e.g., food services—is inadequate or excessive. This know-how is difficult to develop and, in its absence, good budgets are hard to prepare. Decisions on the budgets, at least initially, would need to be based on rough justice. If this approach is taken, there will be complaints that in some cases physicians over whom the hospital has little control are responsible for the cost, and there will be complaints of inequity that one institution is being treated better than another and the complaints will often have merit.

One of the reasons that decisions will be no more than rough is that the data now available are inadequate to support very effective line-item budget review and good data will be expensive and time consuming to obtain, analyze, and use. Even the best data system will have shortcomings. It is likely that budgets will often be padded, and since the existence of padding will be known, it is equally likely proposed budgets will be cut in the review process. The time involved from beginning to end of the process will be long, and there will be a choice sometimes between using outdated information initially collected and delaying the decision. Projections of expected costs will prove wrong because the unexpected—like the current wage and price controls—will sometimes occur.

One issue that is a matter of some controversy is whether, if actual costs were below the budget, the saving would revert to the payors, the hospitals as free money, or whether there would be a sharing of savings. . . .

What I have just been talking about includes many of the nuts and bolts of budget review, and these involve some serious issues and difficulties. But I might conclude by saying that I believe the more important prerequisite for making a hospital budget review and approval system effective is wisdom in the planning of a health system and courage to apply this wisdom. Your decision on whether you would propose to adopt such a system will have to depend on your judgment as to whether this prerequisite will be met.[57]

Because of these problems, officials perceived cost ceilings as the most effective and administratively easiest means of controlling Medicare costs. Ceilings limited costs without requiring detailed regulation of, and conflict with, the health industry. Although the agency had advocated health planning since 1966, BHI officials had little interest or confidence in its effectiveness. Cost limits, in their view, were the "way to go" in cost containment;[58] but they would not have gone this way without legislative support. BHI officials had advocated cost limits for at least three years by the time the amendment was passed, but they had made no move to develop a data system for implementing these limits.[59] In 1972 they started from scratch.[60] Their approach to implementation was as revealing of the balancing strategy as the timing of their action. Because their data were crude, officials said, they set liberal limits on hospital costs, hoping to avoid the "administrative nightmares" of a multitude of hospital appeals. Setting the limit too low initially, said one official, would produce a rash of exceptions and an "administrative mess." Projecting the future of the cost limits provision, BHI officials felt they would have to balance pressure from the hospitals for favorable classifications and limits with budget pressure from the executive branch for lower limits and lower program costs.[61] For the operating officials themselves, this apparently meant balancing their interests in administrative ease and cost containment.

Administrative Changes

While program officials were able to undertake cost limits only with explicit statutory authority, Finance Committee pressure made other administrative actions possible. One was a response to manipulation of accelerated depreciation allowances. BHI presented the problem to HIBAC in May 1969,[62] and the Senate Finance Committee staff addressed it in their February 1970 report.[63] Accelerated depreciation allowed owners to recover investments more rapidly than their property was actually "used up." If they recovered that investment and then reduced or terminated their participation in the program, Medicare paid for a greater share of property depreciation than could be attributed to its use of the property. Furthermore, if the institution were sold, its new owner could repeat the process.

The Senate Finance Committee staff explained the result:

This type of situation could occur where the owner of a property, originally valued at $1 million for purposes of depreciation, sells it for the same amount at the end of 5 years. Assuming a 20-year life on the property, use of the sum-of-the-years digits method of calculating depreciation would yield about 45 percent—or $450,000 in writeoffs during the first 5 years. The new owner, following a brief period of non-participation and reentry into the program, may then proceed to take accelerated depreciation on those same assets, valued at $1 million to him. The property could change hands every few years with the Government eventually paying several times more than the original costs of the assets involved.[64]

A BHI official outlined a similar problem prevalent with Extended Care Facilities (ECFs). Many ECFs were established with Medicare funds. Because they had a high proportion of Medicare patients, Medicare reimbursed them for a major portion of their investment. Reimbursement was calculated on the assumption that the institution would maintain that proportion of Medicare patients for the life of the asset. In fact, however, many ECFs broadened their clientele or left the program, so Medicare was paying these institutions more than its appropriate share of depreciation costs.[65]

In May 1969, BHI proposed to HIBAC a recovery of depreciation reimbursement that exceeded straight-line depreciation where a change in institutional ownership occurred.[66] As described to HIBAC in January 1970, draft regulations apparently addressed only the new owner's depreciation base and not the method of calculation for the new or previous owner.[67] In February, the Senate Finance Committee staff proposed calculating the base for depreciation or asset value differently and eliminating the option to use accelerated depreciation where changes in ownership occurred.[68] In February, SSA's proposed regulation included adjusting depreciation to a straight-line basis when a provider terminated or reduced its participation in Medicare, and further, eliminating the option to use accelerated depreciation on all newly-acquired assets.[69]

The relationship between congressional support and administrative action continued as the proposed regulation was reviewed. The agency received complaints that eliminating accelerated depreciation would interfere with institutions' requirements for cash flow to meet amortization schedules on capital debts—part of the allowance's original justification.[70] The Senate Finance Committee requested a report by the General Accounting Office on hospitals' need for such resources. According to the GAO, SSA had no data on hospitals' use of accelerated depreciation for amortization. Data the GAO compiled indicated that the hospitals' need of accelerated depreciation for that purpose "may not be significant." The GAO therefore recommended that accelerated depreciation not be allowed for any assets, regardless of the date of acquisition.[71]

SSA, said the report, did not want to "disturb any of the options" on assets already acquired.[72] Furthermore, SSA qualified its restriction of the use of accelerated depreciation. They adjusted the regulation to allow accelerated depreciation where cash flow from total depreciation was insufficient to meet an asset's amortization schedule. In such cases accelerated depreciation could not exceed 150 percent of the straight-line rate.[73] BHI officials regarded this limited exception on the one hand as a "relief safety valve" that would seldom be used, and on the other as a constructive response to industry complaints.[74] With this gesture, they appeared responsive to industry without sacrificing their control of abuse. A Ways and Means Committee statement on the issue reinforced their position. Ways and Means cited hospitals' and other institutions' observations that

there is an increasing necessity for health care institutions to finance capital additions through the use of mortgage loans under which, in the absence of accelerated depreciation allowances, they cannot meet the principal amortization schedules they have to pay on capital debts they incur.

In view of this "need," the committee recommended and BHI concurred that accelerated depreciation be allowed for these purposes.[75] By explicitly supporting the exception, the Ways and Means Committee implicitly supported the overall restriction.

This action legitimized using reimbursement to support future capital investment, a policy subject to question in 1966. By 1970, the administration officially advocated reliance on patient revenues instead of government construction grants for capital financing. Based on this premise, the administration advocated substituting a guaranteed loan program for the construction grant program. Although Congress did not agree, their action on accelerated depreciation reinforced this policy position.[76]

BHI officials, however, did not appear concerned with this issue as they changed depreciation regulations. They wanted to eliminate a costly abuse of Medicare reimbursement; the change reduced the availability of accelerated depreciation for noncapital purposes, the use to which it was most likely put. Support from the Ways and Means and Finance committees enabled BHI officials to accomplish their purpose without stormy protest from the industry and its allies. From their balancing perspective, the combination of cost control with political peace was a total success.[77]

Although the change in depreciation regulation affected a reimbursement concession negotiated in 1966, the object of concern was an unintended consequence of the concession rather than the concession itself. In another case—allocation options—the concern was with the concession; that concern arose early in the program and persisted over the years. In May 1969, BHI officials included curtailment of allocation options among the improvements in reimbursement they proposed for HIBAC consideration:

Each hospital has a choice of apportionment procedures which, together with manipulation of charges, may permit an unintended profit. It would seem that all hospitals above a certain size should be required to do departmental accounting and all below that size should be required to use some other approach.[78]

Although they did not include the matter in their February staff report, the Finance Committee addressed the problems presented by allocation options in the February hearings. By that time, the HEW audit agency, the General Accounting Office, and HEW's general counsel had found fault with the impact of the accounting options. The GAO estimated that allowing the combination method added approximately 4 percent to hospital reimbursement under Medicare.[79] In House Government Operations Committee hearings, Committee Counsel Naughton challenged the agency's argument that hospitals lacked the accounting ability for departmental allocation. He cited the GAO's findings (based on fifty-four hospital cost reports) of sufficient data to use either the combination or the departmental method. Each of these hospitals had selected the former, gaining a total of $774,146 over six months. For the first cycle of audited cost reports, which covered one-third of participating hospitals, only 8.2 percent used the departmental RCC method; 44 percent used the combination method with cost finding; 47.2 percent, the combination method with estimates—a temporary option that had ended as scheduled; and 0.6 percent, gross RCC, another temporary option.[80]

None of these challenges outweighed SSA's commitment in 1969 and 1970 not to interfere further in their payment arrangements with hospitals after eliminating the 2 percent plus.[81] Finance Committee persistence, however, ultimately enabled BHI to make the administrative change they had advocated. In December 1970, the Senate Finance Committee included in a report on related legislation a formal recommendation on changes in allocation options. Noting on the one hand that the comptroller general and the HEW audit agency had recommended eliminating the combination method and, on the other, the inability of some institutions to handle the departmental method, the Finance Committee concluded:

It is recognized that medicare cost finding and cost reporting requirements have contributed to an upgrading in recordkeeping and accounting systems, and it does not seem unreasonable now to expect all larger institutions which generally receive larger medical payments to use the more accurate Departmental Method of apportionment between medicare and other payers. On the other hand, the committee is concerned that for smaller providers program cost finding requirements should be simplified wherever possible and wherever equitable.[82]

Following this pronouncement, the Finance Committee staff and BHI agreed on one hundred beds as a dividing line for hospital size. Regulations were changed to require hospitals with more than a hundred beds to use departmental RCC accounting and sophisticated cost finding, and hospitals with less than a hundred beds, the combination method and simplified cost finding. Comments of participating SSA and congressional personnel suggest that this decision balanced accounting precision with political pressure and administrative ease.[83]

In sum, SSA officials recognized excessive payments in the Medicare reimbursement system and believed they should be eliminated. The agency would not act on this, however, without explicit political pressure. Although they acknowledged the usefulness of this pressure, senior officials seemed more resentful of the negative public relations than appreciative of support for the exercise of authority. BHI officials, on the other hand, seemed to welcome congressional advocacy of that authority as an opportunity to control exploitation of the program they ran. Both senior and subordinate officials, however, pressed control only as far as their outside support. In this way, they increased control over program financing with a minimum of political or administrative conflict with the hospitals. Or, more colorfully, they followed a rule attributed to Commissioner Ball: "Screw down, but don't screw up."[84]

Reactions to External Initiatives on Cost Containment

Thus far we have reviewed SSA's goals and strategy through the agency's own initiatives on cost containment. Equally revealing are the agency's responses to the initiatives of others. Where these initiatives were consistent with SSA's desire to restrict payment and would not create political pressure on the agency, SSA's response was enthusiastic. This was true for perhaps the most important cost containment initiative of this period—the Nixon administration's Economic Stabilization Program (ESP). Where an initiative might cut program expenditures but would incur administrative and political costs, SSA assessed the benefits and costs and acted accordingly. On this basis they opposed the budgetary action that eliminated current financing from the reimbursement formula. Two other administration health initiatives, the HMO strategy and beneficiary cost-sharing, conflicted with SSA's cost containment and program agendas. Accordingly, SSA opposed them both. The following account of these developments will therefore demonstrate SSA's political, administrative, and substantive concerns in containing hospital costs.

Economic Stabilization Program

The basic question that ESP raised for Medicare and for the hospitals was whether and how cost reimbursement would be regulated. For hospitals, like other
industries, ESP limited aggregate revenues related to price increases. But prices
or charges constituted less than 50 percent of hospital revenues. If cost reimbursement were not considered a price, more than half the hospitals' revenues
would be immune from controls.[85]

Against the advice of its industry advisory committee and without advance
preparation, in December 1971 the Price Commission simply stated that for
purposes of its regulations, cost was considered a price.[86] This ruling came as a
surprise to BHI as well as to the industry. Three months before, BHI Director
Thomas Tierney had indicated to BHI that because hospital reimbursement was
a cost, the agency believed that cost increases which did not arise from increases
in frozen areas—prices, salaries, and wages—would be allowable in reimbursement.[87] Based on this interpretation, intermediaries were instructed to treat as
"unreasonable," that is, to disallow, any price paid by a hospital that exceeded
a freeze price.[88]

BHI officials perceived the new ruling as an opportunity for far greater control of Medicare reimbursement. Although the Cost of Living Council (CLC) and
the Price Commission had developed limits on aggregate hospital revenues, BHI
officials advocated a limit for each source of revenue, or "class of purchaser."
They reasoned that an aggregate limit of 6 percent, as set by the Council, would
not prevent hospitals from cost reimbursement increases far greater than 6 percent. For example, if a hospital did not raise its charges at all and cost reimbursement constituted half its revenue, it could increase that reimbursement by 12
percent and still be within the overall ceiling. BHI officials were anxious to
prevent this. In February, they presented draft regulations to a staff meeting at
the Cost of Living Council, proposing a 6 percent ceiling on payments from
all classes of purchasers, cost- as well as charge-paying. BHI sent out an intermediary letter with instructions proposed for implementing these limits.[89]

Unfortunately for BHI, the Cost of Living Council did not support this effort to control their program costs. The Cost of Living Council and the Price Commission, supported by the American Hospital Association, reportedly felt that
BHI was usurping their authority.[90] A CLC staff member described BHI's actions
as a "classic case of bureaucracy doing under somebody else's authority what
they couldn't do under their own law." Class of purchaser restrictions, he explained, went beyond CLC authority to limit aggregate increases in revenue.[91] Reinforcing this position were intermediary arguments that BHI's instructions were
excessively burdensome and expensive. The result was a withdrawal of the instructions. The relationship between Medicare and ESP had to be considered anew.

Even if Medicare reimbursement were not explicitly limited under ESP, it
was constrained by the 6 percent ceiling on aggregate revenue increases. Thus the

Medicare system needed ESP rulings on hospital revenues before they could adjust interim payments or make final settlements with the hospitals for a year's costs. After the encounter described above, a BHI official recalled, Medicare officials simply waited for decisions on hospital compliance from ESP officials. But as time passed with no decisions, he explained, hospital cash flow was "drying up" and hospitals began to complain to their congressmen who, in turn, complained to SSA. Accordingly, BHI responded with a new proposal. Unable to establish a ceiling on their costs, they now concentrated on restoring smooth program operations while avoiding overpayment. Their proposal established a mechanism for presumptive hospital compliance with ESP, under which Medicare reimbursement could go forward. Hospitals would be presumed to be in compliance with ESP regulations where the costs presented for reimbursement were less than or equal to 109 percent of the previous year's costs. The 9 percent was the sum of the 6 percent revenue increase which could result from a price change and a 3 percent estimate of increased volume of services. If a hospital's costs exceeded the limit, Medicare would pay up to 109 percent and refer the case to the Internal Revenue Service (IRS). If the IRS indicated that the hospital was in compliance with ESP, Medicare would pay the rest. Thus, IRS, not SSA or its intermediaries, would be the enforcement agency, and this mechanism would protect SSA from overpaying and having to collect.[92]

The mechanism may have served this purpose for SSA but the referral system produced little cost control. Both CLC and BHI officials described IRS as unprepared for these responsibilities and generally ineffective. In fact, a BHI official reported, they rejected the referrals. Again, hospital reimbursement was held up and the hospitals went to their congressmen. SSA then arranged to send IRS a monthly list of hospitals over the limit, leaving IRS to select institutions for investigation. If a hospital were not investigated, SSA would pay whatever the hospitals's costs.[93]

The results from this system were reportedly meager. A CLC staffer felt that any cost control that was accomplished in this period resulted from hospitals' fear and confusion.[94] In any case, according to BHI,[95] if a hospital filed its S-52 ESP compliance form, it got paid. In late 1973, it was decided to eliminate the IRS role; referrals went directly to CLC.

In the meantime, the Price Commission further reduced ESP impact.[96] Institutions whose fiscal years ended after August 1971 had not yet had their interim cost reimbursement rates adjusted when the freeze was instituted. ESP could clearly affect this adjustment, which was generally favorable to providers.[97] BHI recognized the problem for these providers and had included an adjustment factor in their initial control proposal.[98] The Price Commission, however, made a far more expansive ruling—that for hospitals with fiscal years not ended before the freeze, third-party adjustment of reimbursement would disregard ESP, and cost reimbursement base years would be those beginning after the freeze. Thus for the period that its prefreeze fiscal year went beyond August 1972, a hospital's cost reimbursement was not subject to control. This ruling applied to more than three-fourths of the hospitals, a full third of whose fiscal years ran from July 1 to June 30. These were exempt, then, until July 1, 1972.[99] As an HEW-CLC staffer said, this meant a "free ride" for these institutions. For them cost did not constitute a price and thus could be increased, while at the same time the full allowable increase could be put on charge-paying patients.[100] Although the ruling was not put forward until October 1972 and not made final until March 1973, officials felt that it significantly weakened ESP.[101] Concomitantly, it significantly affected Medicare and other third parties.

Throughout ESP's existence, Medicare officials sought to maximize its impact on their program costs. For the most part, they were unsuccessful. Consequently, they concentrated on preventing ESP from disrupting their program operations and on making whatever regulations developed "workable."

Budgetary Action: Eliminating Current Financing

Although "workability" was not an obstacle to measures BHI advocated outside its sphere of political and administrative responsibility, inside it carried greater weight. Within Medicare SSA resisted policy measures that they believed would cost more in program disruption than they would achieve in containing expenditures. One example is their reaction to a 1973 proposal from the Office of Management and Budget (OMB) that advance payments or current financing be eliminated from the Medicare formula. Current financing had been included in reimbursement to ease hospitals' fears about working capital. It consisted of a single payment, adjusted quarterly at first and then biannually, calculated to cover Medicare costs between the time they were incurred by the institution in rendering services and the time the institution received payment for those services. In 1973 these payments were approximately $300 million. SSA believed it incorrect to consider the recall of those funds as a "savings." That $300 million was not a payment that exceeded hospitals' costs; instead it was an interest-free loan. Although recalling the payments would bring $300 million to the federal treasury in one year, leaving it outstanding was costing the government only the interest on that amount. Furthermore, SSA argued, without the payment, hospitals would probably borrow money to cover their working capital needs. Medicare might then have to pay more in reimbursable interest than it had been losing.[102]

SSA took this position even though the General Accounting Office found that many hospitals were investing the Medicare advance rather than using it to pay their bills. "We thought a few hospitals were doing this," reported a BHI official, "but it turned out to be many more."[103] However, SSA felt that the measure's meager results did not warrant disrupting hospital operations and suffering the hospital protest that was bound to result. OMB and the secretary, on the other hand, were impressed by the dollar amounts, and removed current financing despite SSA's protests.

The elimination of current financing was proposed as a regulation in April 1973. Hospitals were to pay it back by June 30, 1973. Given one month for comments on the proposed regulation, the final regulation would leave the hospitals approximately one month in which to return the money. According to a BHI official, 70 percent of the hospitals would have had no problem making the rebate. In this same period, however, hospitals were extremely concerned about controls under ESP and were prevented from increasing their charges. In his view, hospitals viewed the new regulation as "the straw that broke the camel's back."[104] There was consequently an outcry from the industry. As a result hospitals were allowed to pay back the money over a year, and "hardship" cases identified by intermediaries could stretch payment even longer.

The issue did not end there, however. BHI explained to the department that without current financing, the hospitals would flock to periodic interim payment (PIP)—BHI's regularized payment system that most hospitals had not used and which, like current financing, made working capital available. If this occurred, OMB would lose its savings.[105] Consequently, a moratorium was put on PIP until June 30, 1973, while HEW and OMB decided what to do. The issue became how much of an "advance" would be included in PIP—that is, how much time would pass between a hospital's incurrence of an expense and the Medicare payment. Under PIP, the time lag had been 3.5 days.

A BHI official described the two perspectives on the issue.[106] From the budgetary perspective the question was: How can Medicare lose the least interest or lend the least money? The ideal answer would be no advance, or the actual average lag time between expense incurred and payment of a bill—forty-five days. While OMB did not go this far, they advocated a four-week lag.

BHI's perspective and objective were different.[107] They wanted to provide a regular cash flow to the hospitals and to preserve smooth program operations. Accordingly, they believed PIP should approximate the lag between the time an expense was incurred and the time the hospital would have to pay for it. Although this official explained that this gap could not be identified for all expenses, he felt that it could be estimated on the basis of payroll expenditures—usually biweekly. Thus BHI advocated a two-week lag.

In the end, they compromised on a three-week lag. This official observed that the hospitals were better off with the new arrangement than without PIP altogether, but less well off than before the action was taken. Medicare and SSA program arrangements had been disrupted and the hospitals had gotten upset—a result of budget cutting by those who, in the view of SSA officials, lacked concern for program administration.[108]

Alternative Cost Control Strategies

Direct restrictions on hospital payment are not the only way to control hospital revenue. Alternatively, policymakers could encourage market restrictions in two ways. First, they could promote the growth and development of cost-effective medical organizations (health maintenance organizations or HMOs) as competitors of the predominant fee-for-service system. Second, they could increase consumer cost consciousness by increasing the beneficiary's responsibility for medical bills. To avoid excessive burdens, beneficiary cost-sharing could be related to income. Both these approaches to cost containment received considerable attention in the early 1970s and were advocated by the Republican administrations. The Social Security Administration opposed both. Their opposition to financing HMO expansion had much in common with and further explains BHI's advocacy of payment restrictions. Experience had taught BHI officials that excessive payment, once granted, was difficult to recapture. As a result, they approached "innovation" with extreme caution, wary of and anxious to prevent further "rip-offs" of the Medicare program. Opposition to cost-sharing came from a different source—officials' philosophy of social insurance. Both positions add to our understanding of SSA's concerns and commitments in administering hospital insurance.

The HMO strategy turned out to be the Nixon administration's major response to the health care "crisis" they announced in 1969.[109] In 1971 the administration announced as its goal the availability of HMOs to 90 percent of the population by 1980, a qualitative jump from the less than 10 percent at that time enrolled in group practice prepayment plans (GPPPs) on which HMOs were modelled.[110] This strategy first affected Medicare when the administration sought to introduce capitation reimbursement for HMOs under Medicare. SSA had rejected capitation reimbursement for prepaid group practice since the beginning of Medicare, both under regular and experimental authority. As a first step in their HMO activism, in 1970 the administration proposed amending the law to authorize capitation reimbursement specifically. Congress passed such an amendment, called an HMO option. In the amendment's two-year legislative history, however, the Finance Committee continually restricted the payment advantages offered HMOs. The Finance Committee was afraid that the HMO provision

could turn out to be an additional area of potential abuse which might have the effect of increasing health care costs—paying a larger profit than is now or should be paid to these organizations—and decreasing the quality of service available or rendered.[111]

Accordingly, they placed significant constraints on capitation reimbursement.

As finally enacted, established HMOs would receive interim capitation payment, but final reimbursement would be based on the plan's retroactively determined incurred allowable costs. Those costs would be compared to retroactively determined, actuarially adjusted costs of nonmember beneficiaries in the area. Where the plan's costs were lower they would receive a share of the savings, up to a maximum of 7.5 percent of the nonmember Medicare costs. In turn, the government would be responsible for a share of plan costs in excess of nonmember per capita costs, should they occur instead. New HMOs would receive interim capitation payments, retroactively adjusted, with neither rewards nor losses.

This approach eliminated advance capitation and effectively destroyed any encouragement by Medicare of HMO expansion. Reimbursement would be for allowable costs only with no room for financing additional benefits. With regard to the incentives the amendment purportedly intended to present, the final legislation eliminated provision for a government share in the losses, and the reward was not worth to the plans all the additional requirements that the provision placed on an HMO. As a result, two years after the provision's enactment, it was doubtful that Plans would take the option instead of reasonable cost or charge reimbursement.[112]

GPPP lobbyists related the Finance Committee and its staff's attitudes to their experience with the overall program. According to participants, the staff found groups pushing the option to escape existing reimbursement controls. Having just undertaken a major effort to expose the innumerable rip-offs within those controls, the staff's antagonism to more is not surprising. Experience with abuse of capitation in California's Medicaid program reinforced their skepticism.[113] HMO and GPPP advocates, who strongly objected to the option's final form, understood the staff's position. Given the staff's experience with costs exceeding estimates in Medicare as a whole, a GPPP lobbyist suggested, they were understandably wary "of Wilbur Cohens in sheep's clothing."[114]

SSA officials took much the same position as they continued to resist using experimental authority to promote HMO development. According to government advocates of HMOs, who felt that more could be done under that authority,

SSA's attitude is the biggest sticking point. Their concern is that if you open up the trust fund for incentive reimbursement, particularly to develop HMOs, you're opening it up for a real raid.[115]

BHI officials perceived the administration's HMO strategy as a political maneuver glamorizing and distorting a "tired old operation."[116] Partly because of this attitude, responsibility for experimentation was shifted from the policy division of BHI to a separate unit at about this time.[117] But the concerns of operating officials continued to shape experimentation policy. The new experimental division's efforts to establish HMO experiments met the arguments GPPPs had faced five years earlier: HMO control of reimbursement for its beneficiaries would interfere with beneficiary and provider rights, and the availability of data on GPPP performance elsewhere made "experimentation" unnecessary.[118] In response to the argument that a plan's operation on a prepaid capitation basis under Medicare could serve as a prototype for HMO experience under national health insurance, SSA's Office of Research and Statistics questioned whether experimental authority should be used for developmental purposes.[119] As a result, in October 1972 BHI reported to HIBAC:

The HMO experimentation effort which began in June, 1971 was initiated in a climate of high administrative interest and priority. An initial goal was the implementation of six HMO experiments by September 1, 1971. When the HMO option was enacted into law by the passage of H.R.1 and its receipt of Presidential approval on October 30, 1972, no HMO experiments had been put into operation even though HIBAC had given its approval in September to the proposal from Group Health Cooperative in Puget Sound.[120]

BHI officials took an equally cautious position on financing HMO development elsewhere in the department. The question, explained an HEW official, was

whether the HMO strategy should aim towards a goal of having 8 percent of the population enrolled in Kaiser-type organizations, or 92 percent of the population enrolled in "something else" that is a little better than they now have.[121]

Irwin Wolkstein, then BHI deputy director, responded in terms of Medicare experience:

it is not feasible to select, monitor and evaluate a large number—100 or more—highly experimental situations; the level of personnel involved in evaluating potential HMOs will necessarily be not very highly skilled if the workload is large; once you approve an approach because it has turned out badly the chances of getting rid of it are very poor—vested interests develop.[122]

Wolkstein suggested developing criteria for HMO performance, distinguishing between organizations whose experience justified confidence and others for whom experimental arrangements—on which there would be no long-term commitment—were more appropriate.[123]

Interviews revealed further the avoidance of risk and emphasis on control that these comments indicate. Former SSA officials reportedly felt that claims of HMO advantages had been exaggerated and were not being backed by legislative requirements. One official recalled that while HMO advocates argued that competition would make everything "work out," BHI was afraid that the trust fund would be gone before that happened.[124]

SSA's position on cost sharing or copayment had little to do with its commitment to control. I include it here to further elucidate the agency's options and concerns. The administration advocated increased beneficiary copayment in Medicare in 1971.[125] HEW Secretary Elliot Richardson explained their position to the Senate Finance Committee:

We believe that applying coinsurance at an earlier point in a hospital stay will help bring about, at this earlier point, an intensive consideration of whether medically appropriate but less expensive alternatives to hospital care are available.[126]

SSA officials disputed this argument. One explained his point of view. Copayment can be useful, he argued, with services that patients initiate such as physician visits, but it is inappropriate for hospital use, which he considered physician-controlled. While recognizing that studies show a decline in utilization with substantial copayment, he argued that there is no reason to assume that utilization was unnecessary. On the other hand, he believed that the existing deductible offered a savings in program expenditures, while it deterred some misutilization as a by-product and produced only a relatively minor burden on the beneficiary.[127] Because increased cost sharing would conflict with the goal of eliminating financial barriers to care, this official opposed it.

A former HEW official long associated with Medicare also took this position, and explained that existing copayment arrangements in Medicare had nothing to do with market control. Instead, they reflected a "political-psychological" judgment on the acceptable limit of taxation—that is, whatever politicians chose not to tax for, consumers had to pay for.[128]

Proposals to vary copayment with income,[129] intended to prevent creation of financial barriers to necessary care, do not eliminate social insurance advocates' objections. Former officials committed to the Social Security system believe that this introduces an unacceptable means test to a social insurance program. As a former official explained, the payroll tax buys an insurance policy with fixed benefits. To vary those benefits with income means that the same contributions purchase different benefits, thus distorting the contribution-benefit relationship and the perception of contributions as insurance premiums. This official felt that it would transform benefits from a guaranteed right to charity. Once the principle of equal benefits was compromised, taxpayers could not count on where lines would be drawn.[130] Senator Russell Long attributed this point of view to Commissioner Robert Ball. The person who convinced him not to seek income-related copayment, he told his committee, was Bob Ball, who felt that the idea departed too sharply from social insurance principles.[131] Although cost sharing to contain costs was proposed for consideration within the agency[132] and advocated by the administration, it was never encouraged by the Social Security Administration.

Conclusion

SSA's substantive and political strategies for cost containment, which were apparent in the policies they advocated, undertook, and opposed, were directly related to their experience in administering hospital insurance in particular and social insurance in general. Medicare's location in a social insurance program and a social insurance agency placed an overall constraint on cost containment measures. Program designers and administrators perceived Medicare's intent as equal protection of all participants against the costs of illness. Because cost sharing interfered with both protection and equity, social insurance officials found it undesirable.

What SSA considered desirable flowed from its payment responsibility and experience in administering hospital insurance. From the very beginning of Medicare, officials within SSA felt that payment concessions to the hospitals would be inflationary and tried to avoid them, but made these concessions to achieve cooperative working relations with the hospitals. Although some officials perceived these payment decisions as temporary, the agency proved unwilling to risk the political consequences of proposing change. This experience made officials extremely conservative. They resisted innovations like HMOs as new concessions, just as they tried to restrict the concessions already made. At the same time officials showed little interest in detailed involvement in health policy decisions, such as those related to planning and budgeting. In part this stemmed from their general avoidance of political and administrative conflict. But it also seems related to their running a payment program rather than a health program. Although officials recognized that the two were related, their objective was simple and direct control of the payments they made, or a regulatory approach to cost containment.

SSA's equal if not greater commitment to avoiding program disruption and political conflict explains their strategy for achieving their regulatory goals. That strategy was clearly aimed at balancing pressures in the political environment. When SSA was not politically responsible for restrictive action, as with ESP, they advocated strict control. When SSA officials were responsible for the actions they took, they awaited pressure before acting, took advantage of direct congressional support, and went no further than that support extended. Although Congress might have stopped SSA had they attempted more restrictive action, SSA was never prepared to test the limits of its political environment.

SSA's need for hospital cooperation in Medicare implementation might explain its initial political sensitivity. That justification seems less compelling for policy made long after Medicare had become established. Perhaps SSA avoided conflict at least partly because officials did not like it. At least to some extent, a commitment to maintaining smooth operations and administrative peace replaced initial hospital cooperation as an administrative goal. SSA demonstrated this commitment in its response to the elimination of current financing, its implementation of cost limits, and its reactions to the Economic Stabilization Program. Despite officials' desire to control program costs, SSA's cost containment strategy was consistently constrained by their prior commitment to keep Medicare running smoothly.

Notes

1. Although inflation accelerated with Medicare and Medicaid, medical costs rose faster than the overall consumer price index before 1966. For a summary of medical and general inflation rates, see Executive Office of the President, Council on Wage and Price Stability, "The Problem of Rising Health Care Costs," Washington, D.C., April 26, 1976.

2. Karen Davis, "Lessons of Medicare and Medicaid for National Health Insurance," statement prepared for the Hearings of the Subcommittee on Public Health and Environment, Committee on Interstate and Foreign Commerce, U.S. Congress, December 12, 1973, p. 10 (typewritten).

3. Greater costs than estimated also had to do with greater hospital use than anticipated. This summary comes from U.S., Congress, Senate, Committee on Finance, *Medicare and Medicaid: Problems, Issues, and Alternatives*, Report of the Staff to the Committee on Finance, 91st Cong., 1st sess., February 9, 1970, pp. 29-32; U.S., Congress, Senate Committee on Finance, Subcommittee on Medicare-Medicaid, *Medicare and Medicaid: Hearings*, 91st Cong., 2d sess., pp. 27ff.; Robert J. Myers, *Medicare*, published for McCahan Foundation, Bryn Mawr, Pennsylvania (Homewood, Ill.: Richard D. Irwin, Inc., 1970) and addendum, "The Social Security Amendments of 1972" McCahan Foundation, 1973; Robert M. Ball, "Social Security Amendments of 1972: Summary and Legislative History," *Social Security Bulletin* 36 (March 1973): 3-25.

4. The tax for Medicare hospital insurance is 0.9 percent of taxable payroll for employer and for employee. This compares to an overall payroll tax rate of 5.85 percent each.

5. For the structure of Medicare cost sharing, see Myers, *Medicare*, pp. 104-7.

6. *Federal Register*, October 1, 1975, p. 45216.

7. Charles L. Schultze, with Edward K. Hamilton and Allen Schick, *Setting National Priorities; the 1971 Budget* (Washington, D.C.: The Brookings Institution, 1970), p. 76. Unlike Medicare, Medicaid is financed jointly by federal and state government. These expenditure levels represent only the federal share.

8. For a review of medical cost inflation and public policies, see John K. Iglehart, "Explosive Rise in Medical Costs Puts Government in Quandary," *National Journal* 7(September 20, 1975): 1319-28.

9. Schultze, *Setting National Priorities*, pp. 59-60; 1971 budget options are summarized on p. 73.

10. Iglehart, "Explosive Rise in Costs," p. 1319, reprinted with permission.

11. For a review of insurance coverage and gaps, see Karen Davis, *National Health Insurance: Benefits, Costs, and Consequences* (Washington, D.C.: The Brookings Institution, 1975), chapter 3.

12. Politicians from both ends of the political spectrum have withdrawn earlier support for national health insurance because of its inflationary consequences. See, for example, President Gerald Ford, quoted in *National Journal* 8 (January 31, 1976): 135, and Senator John Tunney, excerpts from speech, September 5, 1975, courtesy of the Senator's office. For a review of national health insurance policies in 1975, see Nancy Hicks, "National Health Insurance Now Considered Just Remote Possibility," *New York Times*, December 31, 1975.

13. Schultze, *Setting National Priorities*, p. 73.

14. By this time, HIBAC's influence on policy had declined considerably. Participants and observers attribute the decline to the differences in administrators' needs and interests once the program was under way and to a change in attitudes toward advisory councils with the change in administrations.

15. "Background Material for the Council's Intended Discussion of Medical Costs," Staff Memorandum for HIBAC, HIBAC Agenda Book, January 10-11, 1970.

16. Interview with BHI official.

17. "Control of Medical Costs," Staff memorandum for HIBAC, HIBAC Agenda Book, January 10-11, 1970, pp. 5-6.

18. Ibid., p. 7.

19. Ibid., p. 8.

20. HIBAC Minutes, clearance draft, XXVII, July 19, 1969, p. 14, in HIBAC Agenda Book September 13, 1969.

21. U.S., Congress, House, Committee on Ways and Means, *Medical Care for the Aged: Executive Hearings before the Committee on Ways and Means on H.R. 1 and Other Proposals for Medical Care for the Aged*, 89th Cong., 1st sess., 1965, pp. 783-85.

22. Excerpts from Report of the Committee on Finance, U.S. Senate, to accompany H.R. 6675, p. 36; and excerpts from Report of the Committee on Ways and Means on H.R. 6675, p. 32; both in New Members Background Book, Part I, for HIBAC, 1968.

23. HIBAC Minutes, clearance draft, XXVII, July 1969, p. 14.

24. Interviews with BHI officials.

25. HIBAC, "Control of Medical Costs," pp. 3-4.

26. Ibid.

27. Ibid., and "Suggested Issues for HIBAC Consideration During 1969-70," Staff Memorandum for HIBAC, HIBAC Agenda Book, May 10, 1969, p. 5.

28. "The Nation's Health Care System," Remarks of the President, HEW Secretary Robert H. Finch, Assistant Secretary Roger O. Egeberg, and Undersecretary John G. Veneman on a Report on Health Care Problems and Programs, July 10, 1969, in *Weekly Compilation of Presidential Documents* 5:28, Monday, July 18, 1969, pp. 963-69.

29. Interview with former SSA official involved in legislation.

30. HIBAC Minutes, clearance draft, XXVII, July 19, 1969, pp. 7–9 in HIBAC Agenda Book, September 13, 1969; HIBAC Minutes, XXIX, November 18, 1969, pp. 13–14; U.S., Congress, House, Committee on Ways and Means, *Social Security and Welfare Proposals, Hearings Before the Committee on Ways and Means*, 91st Cong., 1st sess., 1970, p. 133.

31. Committee on Ways and Means, *Social Security and Welfare Proposals*, p. 158.

32. U.S., Congress, Senate, Committee on Finance, *Medicare and Medicaid: Hearings*, 91st Cong., 1st. sess., July 1969, p. 38. The preliminary report focused more on problems with physicians and fiscal agents than with hospitals. Fraud and abuse in the reimbursement of teaching physicians—an area where institutional and physician reimbursement cross—received perhaps the greatest attention.

33. Interviews with committee staff and BHI officials.

34. Committee on Finance, *Medicare and Medicaid: Hearings*, July 1969, p. 381, and *Medicare and Medicaid*, report, February 1970, pp. 45–53.

35. Committee on Finance, *Medicare and Medicaid: Hearings*, February 1970, pp. 73 and 121.

36. Committee on Finance, *Medicare and Medicaid,* report, February 1970, p. 49.

37. Ibid., p. 50.

38. Ibid., pp. 114–16.

39. HIBAC, "Suggested Issues for HIBAC Consideration During 1969–70," May 10, 1969, p. 7.

40. Interview with senior SSA official.

41. Ibid.

42. Interview with former SSA official.

43. Committee on Finance, *Medicare and Medicaid: Hearings*, February 1970, pp. 4ff.

44. See "Statement on the Financial Requirements of Health Care Institutions and Services," Approved by House of Delegates, February 12, 1969, American Hospital Association, and AHA testimony, Committee on Ways and Means, *Social Security and Welfare Proposals*, pp. 1069ff.

45. Irwin Wolkstein, "Overview of Budget Review Systems of Reimbursement," *The Hospital Forum* (December 1972): 11, reprinted with permission.

46. Interviews with BHI officials.

47. Interview with former SSA official.

48. Interview.

49. Interview with senior SSA official.

50. Interview.

51. See U.S., Congress, House, Committee on Ways and Means, *Social Security Amendments of 1970: Report on H.R. 17550*, House Report No. 91-1096, 91st Cong., 2d sess., May 14, 1970, pp. 29–31. The amendments did not actually pass until 1972. See Ball, "Social Security Amendments of 1972." This amendment became P.L. 92–603, Section 222.

52. Committee on Ways and Means, *Social Security Amendments of 1970*, p. 30. The committee went on to express concern that HEW take steps to assure that providers not obtain cost savings by reducing the quality of their care.

53. Interview.

54. HIBAC, "Clarifying the Meaning of Reasonable Cost Under Title XVIII," in HIBAC Agenda Book, March 21–22, 1970, and HIBAC, "Control of Medical Costs," p. 2.

55. See Committee on Ways and Means, *Social Security Amendments of 1970*, pp. 31–35.

56. U.S., Congress, Senate, Committee on Finance, *Social Security Amendments of 1970, Report of the Committee on Finance, to Accompany H.R. 17550*, Senate Report No. 91–1431, 91st Cong., 2d sess., December 11, 1970, p. 121.

57. Irwin Wolkstein, "Overview of Budget Review Systems of Reimbursement," *Hospital Forum* (December 1972): 14, reprinted with permission.

58. Interviews with BHI officials.

59. For a comprehensive review of Medicare's data system and its relative inattention to cost as compared with eligibility data, see Diane Rowland, "Data Rich and Information Poor: Medicare's Resources for Prospective Rate Setting," Harvard University Center for Community Health and Medical Care, Report Series R–45–12, July 1976.

60. Interviews with SSA officials.

61. Interviews with BHI officials.

62. "Suggested Issues for HIBAC Consideration During 1969–70," Staff memorandum for HIBAC, HIBAC Agenda Book, May 10, 1969, p. 5.

63. Committee on Finance, *Medicare and Medicaid*, report, p. 53.

64. Ibid.

65. Interview with BHI official. This problem was probably accentuated by the decline of ECF participation in Medicare related to retroactive claims denial. See chapter 3.

66. HIBAC, "Suggested Issues," p. 5.

67. HIBAC, "Control of Medical Costs," p. 4.

68. Committee on Finance, *Medicare and Medicaid*, report, p. 53.

69. Committee on Finance, *Medicare and Medicaid: Hearings*, February 1970, pp. 169–70. The change also affected the base for calculating reimbursable interest and, to proprietary institutions, return on equity.

70. Interview with BHI officials.

71. U.S., General Accounting Office, *Payments to Hospitals and Extended Care Facilities for Depreciation Expenses Under the Medicare Program*, B–142983, Department of Health, Education, and Welfare, *Social Security Administration*, Report to the Committee on Finance, U.S. Senate, by the Comptroller General of the United States, August 21, 1970, especially pp. 18–21.

72. Ibid.

73. HIBAC minutes, clearance draft, XXXII, May 16, 1970, p. 6, HIBAC Agenda Book, July 24–25, 1970.

74. Interviews.

75. Committee on Ways and Means, *Social Security Amendments of 1970*, pp. 64–65.

76. In fiscal 1968, depreciation paid through Medicare and Medicaid exceeded Hill-Burton funds. See administration testimony, U.S., Congress, House, Committee on Interstate and Foreign Commerce, *Hospital and Health Facility Construction and Modernization, Hearings before the Subcommittee on Public Health and Welfare of the Committee on Interstate and Foreign Commerce*, 91st Cong., 1st sess., March 1969, pp. 22, 31, 36ff., 53–54; and Schultze, *Setting National Priorities*, pp. 60–62.

77. Interviews with BHI officials.

78. HIBAC, "Suggested Issues," p. 5.

79. Committee on Finance, *Medicare and Medicaid: Hearings*, February 1970, p. 73.

80. U.S., Congress, House, Committee on Government Operations, *Administration of Federal Health Benefit Programs, Hearings before a Subcommittee of the Committee on Government Operations*, 91st Cong., 1st sess., p. 46.

81. See chapter 5.

82. Committee on Finance, *Social Security Amendments of 1970, Report on H.R. 17550*, December 11, 1970, p. 179.

83. Interviews with SSA and congressional participants, and HIBAC minutes, clearance draft XXXVII:2, March 27, 1971, p. 15, in HIBAC Agenda Book, April 23–24, 1971.

84. Interview with BHI official.

85. I am indebted for this information and an explanation of its significance to an official serving in HEW and on the staff of the Cost of Living Council.

86. Interviews with BHI and CLC officials.

87. HIBAC minutes, clearance draft, XLII, September 10, 1971, p. 3, in HIBAC Agenda Book, October 15–16, 1971.

88. Interviews with BHI official.

89. Interviews with BHI and CLC officials.

90. Ibid.

91. Interview.

92. Interviews with BHI and HEW-CLC officials.

93. Ibid.

94. Interview.

95. Interview with BHI official.

96. I am indebted to Rob McGarrah, formerly with the Nader Health Research Group, for suggesting investigation of this issue.

97. See Robert E. Schlenker and Richard McNeil, Jr., "Phase II and Phase III Controls on the Hospital Sector," prepared for the staff of the Health Advisory Committee and Cost of Living Council Committee on Health, April, 1973, pp. III-6 and III-7.

98. Interview with BHI official.

99. Schlenker and McNeil, Jr., "Phase II and Phase III Controls," pp. III–6 and III–7.

100. Interview.

101. Interviews with CLC staff; and Schlenker and McNeil, Jr., "Phase II and Phase III Controls," p. III–7.

102. Interviews with SSA officials.

103. Interview.

104. Interview.

105. This account comes from a BHI official.

106. Ibid.

107. Ibid.

108. Ibid.

109. This account comes from interviews with former employees of Interstudy, the consulting firm who, participants say, "sold" the HMO idea to the administration, and from John K. Iglehart, "Health Report/Prepaid Group Practice Emerges as Likely Federal Approach to Health Care," *National Journal* 3(July 10, 1971):1443–52.

110. Ibid., p. 1443.

111. Committee on Finance, *Social Security Amendments of 1970, Report on H.R. 17550*, p. 1320.

112. U.S., Senate, Committee on Finance, *Excerpts from S. Report 92–1230, Report of the Committee on Finance to Accompany H.R. 1, The Social Security Amendments of 1972*, 92d Cong., 2d sess., 1972, pp. 229ff. and interview with official of the Group Health Association of America (GHAA).

113. Interview with congressional participant. See report requested by Chairman Long of the Finance Committee, U.S., General Accounting Office, *Better Controls Needed for Health Maintenance Organizations under Medicaid in California*, B–164031(3), Social and Rehabilitation Service, Department of Health, Education, and Welfare, September 10, 1974.

114. Interview with GHAA official.

115. Official quoted by John K. Iglehart, "Prepaid Group Practices," p. 1449, reprinted with permission.

116. Interview with BHI official.

117. John K. Iglehart, "Prepaid Group Practices," p. 1447, and interview with BHI officials.

118. The arguments were directed at a proposal to pay an advance capitation, at a rate of 80 percent of nonplan Medicare costs, to the Group Health Cooperative of Puget Sound, perhaps the GPPP most highly respected inside and outside BHI. After about a year, suggestions by Ron Carlson in the experimental program led to some adjustments of the original legal opinions, but the experiment continued to encounter obstacles. Enclosure B, "Status of Program Experimentation in the Bureau of Health Insurance," Staff Memorandum for HIBAC, November 28, 1972; and interview with participating BHI official.

119. Interview with BHI official.

120. HIBAC, "Status of Program Experimentation," p. 4.

121. "Meeting on HMO Policy Issues, Baltimore, Maryland, September 17, 1971, p. 1, included in "HMO Policy Issues," Staff Memorandum for HIBAC, HIBAC Agenda Book, October 15–16, 1971.

122. Ibid., p. 2.

123. Ibid., p. 2.

124. Interviews with former SSA officials.

125. According to a former OMB budget examiner, this was an OMB proposal, introduced over the opposition of the department as well as SSA.

126. U.S., Congress, Senate, Committee on Finance, *Social Security Amendments of 1971: Hearings on H.R.1*, 92d Cong., 1st sess., 1971, p. 45.

127. Interview with senior SSA official.

128. Interview. Cf. cost sharing's introduction into Medicare, related to the expansion of hospital days covered, Harris, *A Sacred Trust* (Baltimore, Md.: Penguin Books, Pelican Books, 1969), pp. 196ff.

129. This proposal had to do with National Health Insurance more than Medicare, but is relevant as an option for cost containment.

130. Interviews. Cf. Harris, *A Sacred Trust*, citing Wilbur Cohen, p. 196.

131. U.S., Congress, Senate, Committee on Finance, *National Health Insurance Hearings*, 92d Cong., 1st sess., April 1971, p. 167.

132. In their May 1969 memorandum, "Suggested Issues," for example, BHI officials included the following option: *"Incentives to the Beneficiary*: . . . Another possibility is to apply a daily hospital deductible where a patient enters a hospital which is comparatively high cost . . . for the area."

7

Medicare: The Politics of Federal Hospital Insurance

The Medicare law promised to pay for medical care for the elderly without interfering in its delivery. But this promise ignored a basic economic fact: how care is paid for significantly influences the quantity and quality of care delivered. Thus a payment program necessarily interferes in the practice of medicine. If an agreement to pay for care has no strings attached, it removes any fiscal constraints on physicians' and hospitals' development and delivery of medical services. Alternatively, if the agreement is contingent upon certain conditions, it potentially imposes requirements on professional practice. Legislators thought they had resolved the conflict between promise and reality by requiring conditions on payment, but promising to model them on existing industry practices. In fact, they shifted resolution of the conflict to the bureaucracy, which was left to determine the actual conditions for Medicare payment to hospitals—specifically, which institutions would be paid and how much. How the Social Security Administration made those decisions has been the subject of this study.

SSA could have approached this task in a number of very different ways. They could have dealt with payment issues on a piecemeal, incremental basis, and, as Charles Lindblom suggests, "muddled through."[1] Alternatively, they could have adopted one of two consistent strategies toward program implementation. With a balancing strategy, SSA would make policy choices by identifying relevant political actors, weighing their influence, and compromising their interests to minimize conflict. With a cost-effectiveness strategy, SSA would make policy choices by calculating the most efficient and effective way to finance health services, defining conditions on hospital payment accordingly, and risking conflict to see them observed.

Medicare policy toward hospitals reveals that SSA pursued a balancing strategy of implementation. Medicare officials had devoted enormous time and energy to enactment of federal health insurance over powerful and persistent opposition. In implementation, their primary objective was to ensure the program's success and survival. Although their experience as administrators of social insurance inclined them to avoid involvement in medical practice and to pursue fiscal responsibility, they subordinated both objectives to mobilizing consensus behind Medicare. This task required identifying and satisfying all influential evaluators of Medicare implementation, including beneficiaries who sought care, institutions and professionals who provided it, public health officials who evaluated its quality, and taxpayers—or more directly, congressional tax committees—who paid for it.

The original cornerstone of the balancing process was the Health Insurance Benefits Advisory Council (HIBAC). Composed of representatives of all the constituencies enumerated above, HIBAC's purpose was to arrive at policies these constituencies would accept and to assure their acceptance through policy development. To achieve these goals, SSA substantially reversed the advisory relationship. Rather than take the council's positions as recommendations for government decisions, SSA officials presented their own positions as recommendations to the council. Regardless of officials' preferred course of action, they adapted their policies to reflect the council consensus. Thus, on quality enforcement, where SSA was reluctant to act, they accepted HIBAC recommendations for promulgating uniform and relatively high standards for hospital participation. With reimbursement, on the other hand, BHI modified its commitment to payment control to reflect the council's consensus behind financing hospital maintenance and expansion.

In achieving consensus, the council did more than add up participants' interests. Because members were chosen as individuals and were not officially responsible to the interest groups with which they were affiliated, they could reject or mediate special interest demands. Thus HIBAC rejected a physician consultant group's demand that SSA avoid case-by-case utilization review and state agency involvement; produced a compromise among hospitals, public health professionals and SSA on hospital quality standards; and substantially, though not completely, reconciled the industry's and the health community's interest in generous reimbursement with congressional spending limitations. With these actions, the council served both as a forum for compromise and a source of legitimacy for SSA policy. When HIBAC resisted an interest group representation, SSA generally felt able to do the same.

SSA's concern with consensus shaped initial policy outcomes as well as the policy process. SSA's first responsibility in hospital policy was to implement the law's requirement that hospitals meet minimum quality standards to receive Medicare funds. Specifically, the question was what requirements to impose on the many small institutions that could not meet the industry's own standard of hospital quality. SSA's answer reflected its commitment to public acceptance of Medicare and to political consensus as the means to achieve it. For officials from President Johnson to SSA's Bureau of Health Insurance (BHI), successful implementation depended above all on the availability of a Medicare-financed bed to anyone seeking care on the program's first day. Because of uncertainty as to how many beneficiaries would seek care, sheer numbers dictated liberal requirements for hospital quality. However, SSA's interest in liberal certification went beyond numbers, to satisfying what they perceived as the elderly's and the nation's expectations for Medicare performance—that hospital services be covered where people generally received them. Stringent requirements for Medicare participation could potentially disrupt existing patterns of use and delivery of hospital services, disappointing the elderly and antagonizing the hospitals. On the other hand, public health professionals in the bureaucracy and on HIBAC believed that institutions unable to meet certain structural requirements were unfit to deliver care.

To achieve support from all influential interests, SSA sought to compromise them. Thus they promulgated uniform and relatively high quality standards, satisfying quality advocates, and developed a flexible measure of compliance that enabled them to certify almost all the nation's hospitals. This solution had the additional advantages to SSA of avoiding administrative problems with multiple sets of standards and rigid measures of compliance, and of facilitating quiet desegregation of the nation's hospitals, a secondary but important goal for Medicare officials.

When it came to implementing the law's requirement that participating hospitals establish physician committees to review hospital use, SSA's strategy of compromise and consensus was equally apparent. These utilization review committees did not exist in most hospitals before Medicare, leaving SSA to oversee development of a new professional practice. Because HIBAC did not debate this issue, there is no direct evidence of the process of compromise and consensus behind SSA's decisions. Its substance, however, is apparent in a comparison of actual policy with interests articulated by affected parties. One of these was Congress. Despite the quality assurance and cost containment that utilization review theoretically entailed, cost concerns were the primary reason for requiring utilization review in Medicare. SSA, supported by HIBAC, reflected this concern by rejecting AMA demands that utilization review not be used to determine payment. SSA, with equal support from HIBAC, nevertheless made policy responsive to both organized medicine's and organized hospitals' opposition to government control over medical practice. Thus SSA established only minimal requirements for the review process, limited governmental (state agency) responsibility for overseeing utilization review to those minimal requirements, delegated responsibility for overseeing utilization review performance to private agents (primarily Blue Cross plans) that lacked enforcement authority but had established cooperative relations with the hospitals, and generally encouraged rather than enforced compliance with the law.

Officials explained these policy decisions primarily in terms of the administrative convenience of letting hospitals shape their own review processes and of relying on the claims-paying agents who were most ready and willing to oversee them. But the consistency of administrative convenience with non-interference in professional practice reflected officials' conception of Medicare as a program of claims payment more than delivery of care, and inclination toward conciliation of the most alert and powerful affected interest—professional and institutional providers of care.

SSA's payment compromise differed somewhat from its quality compromise. Officials within SSA had substantive objectives for payment, notably accuracy and control, that they lacked on quality issues. Had they pursued these objectives, or compromised them on grounds of technical feasibility, we might conclude that SSA pursued a cost-effectiveness strategy. In fact they compromised those objectives to conciliate the hospitals and achieve a political consensus. More specifically, SSA liberalized accounting requirements to mitigate hospital fears more than to adjust to their technical capacities, liberalized capital payments to reflect a consensus on Medicare's financing obligations to which BHI officials did not subscribe, and went beyond the consensus with concessions to appease the hospital industry. These concessions nevertheless fell significantly short of hospital demands, because SSA was equally concerned with potential congressional opposition to payment arrangements that would require tax increases. Although elements of BHI's commitment to accurate and controlled payment remained in the reimbursement formula, SSA's final policy rested primarily on its compromise of hospitals' interest in maximum reimbursement with congressional reluctance to raise taxes.

With this compromise, Medicare officials intended to achieve more than hospital willingness to accept Medicare patients. Officials believed that the hospitals would have done this much on less favorable terms, but reluctant participation did not satisfy their goal of supportive consensus. To achieve it they made policy that turned hospitals from adversaries into allies in Medicare implementation.

SSA's balancing strategy for implementation achieved its primary objective: acceptance of federal health insurance in American society. Given the controversy that preceded Medicare's enactment, this was no small task. The administrative effort and skill involved in developing the consensus we have examined, not to mention that required in managing the eligibility, record-keeping and bill-paying process, was enormous. To program administrators, this achievement was worth the initial departure from both their own objectives for payment control and others' goals for hospital quality. Furthermore, Medicare administrators did not consider their initial decisions on quality and payment necessarily permanent. Consistent with their strategy of compromise, they considered them reflections of the contemporary political climate, adjustable as the climate changed.

While adjustment did in fact occur, this perspective underestimated the lasting impact of their initial compromises and the strategy's tendency toward entrenchment rather than adaptation. Without reevaluating the necessity or desirability of initial policies, SSA generally avoided action that would disrupt the substantive, political and administrative compromises of 1965–1966. In other words, maintaining the initial compromises they made to ensure survival became SSA's definition of administrative success once they achieved survival.

Despite general recognition that Medicare had certified hospitals with health and safety violations, SSA maintained its initial compromise on quality with an "educational" rather than an enforcement approach to quality standards. To terminate a noncomplying hospital's participation, SSA required lengthy and time-consuming documentation of both a hospital's deficiencies and state agency consultation to correct them, proceeded only when that documentation produced an unassailable legal case, and then acted in close consultation with the affected congressional representatives. In this way SSA continued to balance the pressure they perceived from hospitals and their communities to maintain Medicare financing with pressure from health professionals to improve hospital quality. As a result, Medicare continued to support unsafe and inadequate hospitals.

SSA believed this approach the best way to improve hospital quality in a political environment. But their satisfaction with the approach, and the compromise of interests behind it, made them unresponsive to alternatives that could have altered the environment. Publicly proposed alternatives included public disclosure of SSA's hospital surveys and elimination or adjustment of the medicare law's delegation of certification responsibility to the industry's Joint Commission on Hospital Accreditation. Both proposals would have expanded the pressures SSA faced. Public disclosure would have transformed SSA's certification activity from a private professional exchange between surveyors and the hospital to a publicly visible process, and could have reduced beneficiaries' ignorance or unconcern about quality, on which SSA's existing compromise was based. The result would be a new source of pressure in the certification process. Similarly, if SSA became responsible for certifying all hospitals, not simply unaccredited ones, the pressures it faced would expand accordingly. Although willing to compromise on the second proposal, SSA reacted to both measures as unwelcome disruptions of comfortable arrangements. In making this judgment, they failed to recognize that their restriction of public responsibility reinforced a distribution of power they had only intended to reflect.

SSA's initial approach to utilization review also established an administrative framework and perspective that shaped later policy. From the beginning SSA avoided enforcing a qualitative review process, treated utilization review as an audit of claims payment rather than of professional practice, and relied on claims reviewers or intermediaries to monitor utilization review committee performance. When use of Extended Care Facilities beyond Medicare's intentions posed a fiscal problem, SSA saw action through the claims process—that is, retroactive denial—as most appropriate, rather than reassessment or enforcement of utilization review. Furthermore, when the Senate Finance Committee proposed to establish a new quality and fiscal review mechanism, the Professional Standards Review Organization (PSRO), SSA opposed it as a disruption of the payment control mechanism they had established, which would entail an involvement in professional practice they had managed to avoid.

When it came to payment, SSA perceived the initial arrangements as a good compromise between congressional and hospital interests and were anxious to maintain it. Further concessions to the hospitals conflicted with the bureaucracy's own commitment to payment control and could antagonize the Congress;

payment restrictions would arouse the relatively latent hospital pressure for more liberal payments. SSA's preoccupation with this political compromise meant unwillingness to adjust reimbursement for providers with little political influence, like prepaid group practices; conciliation of public concern about rising costs with token experimentation that attempted little and risked nothing; and protection of commitments made to the hospitals in the 1965–1966 agreement. As long as the initial deal with the hospitals posed fewer political risks than did change, SSA showed little interest in evaluating hospital reimbursement in light of rampant hospital cost inflation. Hence the original payment arrangements became entrenched as SSA's standard of payment adequacy or "fairness," independent of their impact or appropriateness.

This occurred despite continuing concern on the part of some SSA officials that the facts did not justify those payment arrangements. Aware that hospital reimbursement in excess of costs fueled hospital expenditures and raised hospital costs, these officials wanted to restrict payments they considered excessive. This concern did not outweigh the agency's commitment to political peace, and in the absence of political pressure, SSA limited its restrictive actions to the relatively uncontroversial area of manipulation of reimbursement for unintended purposes, notably personal gain. But in contrast to other policy areas, officials' interest in cost containment led them to welcome rather than resist political pressure for further action. Thus they responded to criticism from the powerful Senate Finance Committee with restrictions on reimbursement which they had previously considered but had been slow or unwilling to undertake, including support for legislation to establish "reasonable" limits on individual hospital reimbursement, restrictions on accelerated depreciation, and withdrawal of allocation options.

While SSA's responsiveness to political pressure on cost containment differed from its posture on quality, the agency continued to assess political pressure and to avoid conflict and disruption. They minimized political disruption by culling powerful external support for each restrictive measure, moving no further than that support extended, and minimized administrative disruption by slow and cautious implementation of the measures they adopted.

Similarly, when it came to the cost containment proposals of others, SSA reflected both their interest in cost containment and their reluctance to incur political or administrative disruption to achieve it. Thus officials first welcomed the Economic Stabilization Program (ESP) as an opportunity to contain Medicare costs while someone else suffered the political heat. When ESP officials rejected this interpretation of their mandate, SSA officials directed their attention instead to mitigating ESP's disruption of Medicare's payment process. Within their own program, SSA opposed budgetary measures like the removal of current financing, which would save little in program expenditures but would interfere with existing hospital cash flow and therefore program operations. When it came to assessing Health Maintenance Organizations (HMOs), officials responded in terms of their political experience. They had learned that payment commitments once made were politically difficult to retract; therefore the way to contain costs was to avoid new commitments and restrict existing ones as politically feasible. Committed to this regulatory strategy for cost containment, SSA officials opposed the market-improvement approach offered by HMOs. To BHI officials, payment rules that encouraged HMOs would offer one more opportunity for exploiting the Medicare trust fund; their desire to prevent further waste made them distrust innovation.

In sum, SSA's initial goal in Medicare implementation was to secure the program's success and therefore its survival; the means to achieve it were political compromise and consensus. The strategy was eminently successful in getting Medicare under way and accepted. But in the process, maintaining the compromises through which the goal was achieved became an end in itself. If Medicare officials can be criticized, it is less for the compromises they made in the name of survival than for their failure to reevaluate them as time passed and circumstances changed.

Basically, SSA had a mission to perform: to establish federal payment for medical care as acceptable in American society. Once that mission was accomplished, officials had no desire to solve the problem it had exacerbated in the nation's health care system. Despite changes in the political environment, suggested by enactment of the PSRO legislation and consumer law suits on certification, SSA had no interest in exercising authority over professional practice. Even on costs, where officials did have an interest in greater authority, they directed their efforts to control of their own program more than to broad solutions of medical care delivery problems to which Medicare contributed. Although SSA may have avoided involvement in health policy as a strategy for achieving the long-term goal of national health insurance, officials' explanations of policy suggest that their basic motivations were more immediate: essentially their satisfaction with their task as they had defined and implemented it and aversion to the conflicts inherent in change. The result is an inherent bias toward the interests that initially dominated policy even after survival has been secured, rather than a continuing adaptation to a shifting political environment.

In the choices posed and the strategy for resolution, SSA's implementation of Medicare had much in common with the United States Office of Education's (OE's) handling of the Elementary and Secondary Education Act (ESEA).[2] Enacted in the same year, both laws initiated major federal intervention in a sphere where it had long been resisted; both entailed payments to independent actors—state and local education authorities in the one case, hospitals in the other—to deliver services to a specified population; both left administrators to reconcile conflicts between federal responsibility and "noninterference"; and both were administered by agencies primarily concerned with getting their program under way. Although ESEA promoted educational reform, in contrast to Medicare's commitment to the status quo, a noninterference clause, congressional support for state and local autonomy, and administrative conservatism substantially reduced this difference.

With similar environments, tasks, and administrative objectives, the agencies pursued similar strategies. In their study of ESEA implementation, Bailey and Mosher characterize OE's task:

to define the options available to the State educational agencies and/or the local educational agencies, or other grantees, and to deal with the technical and political dilemmas posed by the statute in ways that would be likely to enlist the understanding, concurrence, and enthusiasm of these partner-clients.[3]

Like the hospitals, those "partner-clients" saw an opportunity in the availability of federal funds to pursue their own ends, which departed significantly from the legislation's intent. Accordingly, "hope, anxiety, uncertainty, inexperience, and fear at the local level comprised the intellectual and emotional setting"[4] for program implementation.

The process through which OE assuaged those fears was one of continual consultation and compromise with affected interests. Professional staff proposed restrictive guidelines that were adjusted and withdrawn under pressure; requirements were minimized under "pressure of time"; an enormous public relations effort was mounted; and a sympathetic relationship was established with state and local education authorities.[5] Like SSA and Medicare, OE tried to turn states and localities from adversaries to allies in program implementation.

Avoiding conflict with institutions on which federal agencies depend but which they do not control is characteristic of a broad range of programs. The Department of Housing and Urban Development has ignored illegal racial discrimination to avoid alienating local supporters of its public housing program;[6] the federal public assistance agency has placed few substantive requirements on state welfare programs.[7] Even where agencies do not avoid conflict initially, their willingness to engage in confrontation declines over time. Interestingly enough, SSA's predecessor, the Social Security Board, illustrates this pattern. Although they were initially aggressive in asserting control over the states' administration of the public assistance program,

the intensity of federal control of the public assistance program probably diminishes as the federal agency responsible for administration becomes less insecure, less of a novelty, and begins to establish quiet negotiation procedures that could serve as alternatives to noisy withdrawal of federal cooperation. In other words, as the federal agency grows older, it can be expected to be more likely to establish an accommodation with its clientele group—in this case, the state public assistance policy-makers.[8]

Whether from their inception or later in life, government agencies tend to pursue stable working relations with other political actors. Administrators become committed to preserving those relationships despite their unsuitability for new tasks or for fiscal control. The Office of Education, for example, was a service organization which provided data and technical assistance to the states before it became responsible for overseeing state and local use of federal funds. Developing criteria for grants and monitoring compliance were tasks for which it had no experience. Although the agency acquired new leadership and was totally reorganized in 1965, OE performed its new tasks from its traditional perspective of service and technical assistance rather than from a new perspective of leadership and oversight.[9]

In assessing ESEA's impact on a local school system, Mark Arnold observes:

Title I can best be viewed as a vast funding machine. Congress grinds out money. The Office of Education funnels it to the states according to formula. As long as the formula is followed, the people who run the machine are satisfied. More and more money siphons into local districts each year. The trouble with the system is there is no incentive to produce, and no penalty for failure to produce. The only pressure is to spend the money, in as many schools as the law will allow.[10]

Through the 1960s, OE officials generally avoided responsibility for monitoring and evaluation. To illustrate administrators' attitudes, Jerome Murphy quotes an OE official:

Other than making sure states got their money and making sure it was spent, there was no role for the Office of Education. I don't know anyone around here who wants to monitor. The Office of Education is not investigation-oriented, never has been, and never will be.[11]

Furthermore, OE did not follow through on the law's explicit requirement that it evaluate the effectiveness of ESEA expenditures:

Since the beginning of the program, evaluation has been high on the list of federal rhetorical priorities, but low on the list of actual USOE priorities. The reasons for this are many. They include fear of upsetting the federal-state balance, recognition of that [sic] little expertise exists at the state and local levels to evaluate a broad-scale reform program, and fear of disclosing failure. No administrator is anxious to show that his program is not working.[12]

As these observations suggest, OE's reluctance to lead and monitor state and local authorities through the 1960s resulted from several factors, notably a predisposition toward its traditional role and a rational calculation of the political benefits of the status quo versus the costs of change. States and localities, supported by their congressmen, provided the most active and consistent pressure on ESEA administrators. To the extent that OE sought certain objectives, it therefore used encouragement to achieve them, ignored noncompliance and did not terminate a grant.[13] Martha Derthick describes similar behavior in the federal administration of public assistance in Massachusetts. Although the federal agency seems to have exerted more leadership than OE, cooperative relationships were established, noncompliance with administrative requirements tolerated, and termination of grants not seriously considered.[14]

Satisfaction with the procedures and relationships they have established sometimes makes federal agencies unresponsive to changes in the political environment. Rather than accommodate new political actors or pressures, they ally with the actors whom they theoretically oversee to protect arrangements from disruption. For example, OE supported state and local agencies in resisting demands for new directions in funding from newly organized welfare mothers. Allied with state and local agencies, OE perceived the welfare mothers' demands "as a threat to Title I's 'integrity' and the whole operation as a 'raiding party.'" Committed to their "primary constituency"—the public school system through which they worked—OE was unresponsive to what might be considered its more appropriate constituency, "the poor people whose children the legislation is supposed to assist." As a result, OE was overruled by the secretary of HEW.[15]

Where federal agents are dissatisfied with existing arrangments, however, a change in the environment can provide an opportunity for action. In OE, as in SSA, federal officials have sometimes favored action that states and local education agencies opposed. Most often, they have been unsuccessful; guidelines have been "sent up," but at some level of decision they have been modified or withdrawn "under political pressure."[16] On one occasion, Jerome Murphy explains, the obstacles to action were overcome. From the beginning of the program, OE officials had advocated parent involvement in ESEA funded programs and proposed the development of appropriate requirements. Such requirements were successfully opposed by the state and local agencies until OE was subject to counterpressure by a lobby for the poor. With the presence of organized pressure to do what they wanted to do, OE was able to institute the require-ments they had long advocated.[17]

Perhaps even more significant, pressure can sometimes produce organizational change. In the early 1970s, public criticism led a new administration to try to change ESEA implementation. Reorganization, new staff positions, aggressive leadership and executive support meant new organizational attitudes and a new environment, and OE undertook a major effort in management and enforcement, which it had previously avoided. After a brief period, however, public pressure and executive support declined, and the agency tended toward stability and peace in its relations with the states.[18]

The experiences of SSA and similar agencies reveal federal agencies seeking to gain support and overcome threats within their environments; achieving stable relations with relevant political actors; avoiding disruption of those relations in directions they oppose; and shifting those relations in directions they favor only with visible external support. Although transformations in these relations occur, they seem dependent both on changes within the bureaucracy and on persistent external pressure. This pattern is consistent with some general propositions about bureaucratic behavior.

First is the agency's need for political support. Anthony Downs begins his analysis of bureaucracy with the premise that

no bureau can survive unless it is continually able to demonstrate that its services are worthwhile to some group with influence over sufficient resources to keep it alive.[19]

Conversely, one might say that no bureau or program can survive unless it reconciles those groups with influence over sufficient resources to destroy it. In combination, the two principles led SSA to accommodate several political actors in its initial implementation of Medicare. Pressure from those actors has not been equal, however, and policy has tended to reflect the interests of the hospital industry. While the industry's assertion of its interests has been constant, assertion of other interests has been intermittent or limited. This has happened because Medicare payments impose what James Q. Wilson has termed "concentrated costs and distributed benefits." The hospital industry and medical profession, who benefit from maximum payment with minimum control, constitute a "sector of society conscious of its special identity," and therefore readily mobilized for political action to protect its interests. Acquiescing in those interests imposes costs, primarily in rising medical expenditures and taxes without regard to the health benefits derived. But those costs are widely distributed over a "large, diverse group" of consumers and taxpayers, "with no sense of special identity and no established patterns of interaction." Hence they are less likely, or more difficult, to mobilize for political action.[20] Costs do become concentrated for congressional committees who wish to have popular programs and avoid raising taxes, and they have therefore challenged hospital interests. But congressmen too feel disproportionate pressure from the industry and the public at large, and often acquiesce in the industry's interests.

Faced with this configuration of pressures, SSA's quest for survival required above all conciliation of the hospital industry. Although policy took quality control and limited revenue into account, administrators concentrated on establishing workable relations with the hospitals. Once procedures and relationships were established, SSA manifested a second characteristic of bureaucratic behavior: a bias toward preserving the status quo. As Anthony Downs has observed:

Like most large organizations, bureaus have a powerful tendency to continue doing today whatever they did yesterday. The main reason for this inertia is that established processes represent an enormous previous investment in time, effort, and money. This investment constitutes a "sunk cost" of tremendous proportions. Years of effort, thousands of decisions (including mistakes), and a wide variety of experiences underlie the behavior patterns a bureau now uses. Moreover, it took a significant investment to get the bureau's many members and clients to accept and become habituated to its behaviors.

If the bureau adopts new behavior patterns, it must incur at least some of these costs all over again. Therefore, it can rationally adopt new patterns only if their benefits exceed both the benefits derived from existing behavior and the costs of shifting to the new patterns.[21]

In essence, "sunk costs" mean that bureaucracies need a reason to change. What constitutes a reason has to do with political environment and administrators' predispositions. Short of a threat to its survival, a bureaucracy has leeway in responding to changes in the political environment. It can ignore them, resist them, or use them to its own ends. SSA's political environment has changed since 1965. Although the medical industry remains the most powerful actor, it no longer poses a threat to Medicare's survival. Furthermore, challenges to industry interests from both Congress and the executive branch, though limited, have provided some support for a greater exercise of government authority. SSA's responses to these changes have been cautious and selective, reflecting both its calculations of the political costs of change versus the benefits of the status quo and its ideological predispositions.

On quality, challenges to SSA's policy of nonintervention have come from the Congress, for example, in its enactment of PSROs, and from consumer advocates, through the courts. SSA has not responded. The reason has much to do with what Herbert Kaufman has called "tunnel vision:"

Organization leaders and members who seem to be unaware of transformations that are conspicuous to others are not wanting in intelligence, humanity and good intentions. They slip into their unyielding ruts by imperceptible stages because their attention is so totally concentrated on the specialized functions that must be completed day by day if the output of their organization is not to cease altogether.

After some years of all these pressures, both unconscious and deliberate, an organization's policies and procedures are apt to become for many people, including (indeed, perhaps especially) those at high level, the natural, automatic ways of acting. Not only are they *disturbed* by suggestions that change is required; they are *astounded* because any other pattern is unimaginable.[22]

Medicare was designed and implemented by social insurance professionals as a program for claims payment more than health care delivery. From the beginning SSA officials perceived quality control as a constraint more than an objective in providing social insurance benefits. Reinforcing their calculations of the political risks of government oversight of professional practice were a preoccupation with claims payment and a general lack of experience and interest in quality control. Thus, while SSA responded to pressure from public health professionals, they avoided enforcing institutional standards and substituted controlling claims for overseeing medical practice. Once they established this modus vivendi, SSA officials were relatively comfortable and were both disturbed and astounded by proposals for change. Accordingly, they continued to find claims control preferable to professional oversight, and opposed PSROs; objected to major changes in their responsibility for institutional certification; and resisted publicity and consumer involvement in the certification process. This behavior was as much a product of "tunnel vision" as of political calculations.

On costs, SSA behaved somewhat differently. From 1965, officials within SSA sought accuracy and control in paying the hospitals and were critical of compromises made to conciliate the industry. Their criticism was a necessary but not a sufficient condition for a change in policy. As Downs had observed:

No bureau will alter its behavior patterns unless someone believes that a significant discrepancy exists between what it is doing and what it "ought" to be doing.[23]

But once a "performance gap" is perceived,

the second step in changing bureau behavior consists of the process of communication and persuasion through which the officials who initially perceive a significant performance gap convince others that it exists, and that something ought to be done about it.

But even this step will not change the bureau's behavior unless the group of officials who are convinced that something ought to be done includes those who have the power and authority to do it.[24]

On cost containment, senior officials were not convinced until the powerful Senate Finance Committee—perhaps encouraged by frustrated bureaucrats—publicly expressed the criticisms that had been ignored within the agency. A desire to respond to congressional critics then overcame senior officials' preoccupations with existing arrangements. Congressional support also reduced the risk of political conflict that they associated with change. Hence senior officials were prepared to take action they had previously rejected, and SSA gradually increased its control over hospital payment.

But here too change was limited by ideological predisposition as well as political calculations. "Tunnel vision" committed SSA to regulation as the only way to achieve cost containment. They found consumer cost sharing inconsistent with their social insurance principles, and innovation likely to exploit the trust fund. Perhaps even more important, SSA perceived medical cost inflation less as an indication of poor performance in Medicare administration than as an unfortunate concomitant of their successful claims-paying program. Although they were prepared to exert gradual control over their own program costs, they found the responsibility for restructuring the medical market largely outside their purview.

Though perhaps disappointing, SSA's perspective is not surprising. Unlike many other federal programs,[25] Medicare has not failed to fulfill its legislative promise; rather it has failed to tackle the problems that fulfillment has raised. The lesson of Medicare is that a bureaucracy charged with and experienced in the payment of claims will have limited interest in confronting the health cost and quality problems to which third-party claims payment leads. To ensure program survival in a hostile environment, SSA made compromises that perpetuated inadequate and unsafe institutions and exacerbated medical cost inflation. Like numerous other organizations and bureaucracies, it became committed to the compromises it had worked long and hard to achieve. Both ideological predisposition and aversion to political risk made SSA comfortable with the status quo and resistant to change. To change Medicare policy, it is therefore necessary to alter both administrators' predispositions—for example, through changes in personnel and organization—*and* the risks they face in change versus the status quo. Responsibility for altering the course of Medicare policy or any expansion of federal health insurance therefore rests less with administrators than with the Congress and the executive to which they are responsible.

Notes

1. Charles E. Lindblom, "The Science of Muddling Through," *Public Administration Review* 19(1959): 79–88.

2. This description of ESEA implementation is based on Stephen K. Bailey and Edith K. Mosher, *ESEA: The Office of Education Administers a Law* (Syracuse, New York: Syracuse University Press, 1968); Jerome T. Murphy, "Title I of ESEA: The Politics of Implementing Federal Education Reform," *Harvard Educational Review* 41 (February 1971):35–63, copyright 1971 by the president and Fellows of Harvard College; and Jerome T. Murphy, "The Education Bureaucracies Implement Novel Policy: The Politics of Title I of ESEA, 1965–72," in Allan P. Sindler, ed., *Policy and Politics in America* (Boston: Little, Brown, 1973), pp. 160–198.

3. Bailey and Mosher, *ESEA*, p. 99.

4. Ibid., p. 101.

5. Ibid., chapter 4. Unlike early Medicare implementation, when Congress was considered more than consulted, congressmen played an active role in evaluating ESEA guidelines. In further contrast, congressional interest supported more than countered the interests of independent actors, that is, state and local education agencies.

6. See Frederick Aaron Lazin, "The Failure of Federal Enforcement of Civil Rights Regulations in Public Housing, 1963–1971: The Cooptation of a Federal Agency by its Local Constituency," *Policy Sciences* 4(1973): 263–73.

7. See Martha Derthick, *The Influence of Federal Grants* (Cambridge, Massachusetts: Harvard University Press, 1970), particularly pp. 195ff., on constraints on federal objectives for state and local action; and Gilbert Y. Steiner, *Social Insecurity: The Politics of Welfare* (Chicago, Illinois: Rand McNally and Co. 1966), especially pp. 243ff.

8. Steiner, *Social Insecurity*, p. 84.

9. Jerome T. Murphy, "Title I of ESEA," pp. 40ff.

10. Mark R. Arnold, "Public Schools," in Sar A. Levitan, ed., *The Federal Social Dollar in Its Own Back Yard* (Washington, D.C.: The Bureau of National Affairs, Inc., 1973), p. 45.

11. Jerome Murphy, "Title I of ESEA," p. 42, reprinted with permission.

12. Ibid., p. 43, reprinted with permission.

13. For a comprehensive analysis, see Jerome Murphy, "Title I of ESEA," especially pp. 44–46.

14. See Martha Derthick, *Federal Grants*, chapter 8, especially p. 208.

15. Jerome Murphy, "Title I" pp. 50–51, reprinted with permission.

16. Ibid., pp. 46–51, reprinted with permission.

17. Ibid., pp. 46–48, and, on usefulness of "countervailing power," pp. 61–62.

18. See Jerome T. Murphy, "The Education Bureaucracies," pp. 184ff.

19. Anthony Downs, *Inside Bureaucracy* (Boston: Little, Brown, 1967), p. 7.

20. See James Q. Wilson, "The Politics of American Business Regulation," in James McKie, ed., *Social Responsibility and the Business Predicament,* (Washington, D.C.: The Brookings Institution, 1974), pp. 135–168.

21. Downs, *Inside Bureaucracy*, p. 195. Downs attributes assertion of the "'sunk costs' doctrine" to J.G. March and H.A. Simons, *Organizations,* (New York: Wiley, 1958), p. 173.

22. Herbert Kaufman, *The Limits of Organizational Change* (University, Alabama: The University of Alabama Press, 1971), p. 21. Emphasis in original.

23. Downs, *Inside Bureaucracy*, p. 191.

24. Ibid., p. 194.

25. For studies of programs that government could not implement, see Martha Derthick, *New Towns In-Town* (Washington, D.C.: The Urban Institute, 1970); and Jeffrey C. Pressman and Aaron Wildavsky, *Implementation* (Berkeley, California: University of California Press, 1973).

Selected Bibliography

Books

Bailey, Stephen K., and Mosher, Edith K. *ESEA: The Office of Education Administers a Law*. Syracuse, N.Y.: Syracuse University Press, 1968.

Briloff, Abraham J. *Unaccountable Accounting*. New York: Harper and Row, 1972.

Brown, J. Douglas. *An American Philosophy of Social Security: Evolution and Issues*. Princeton, N.J.: Princeton University Press, 1972.

Brown, William G.; Harbison, Frederick H.; Lester, Richard A.; and Somers, Herman M., eds. *The Princeton Symposium on the American System of Insurance: Its Philosophy, Impact, and Future Development*. Held June 1967. New York: McGraw-Hill, 1968.

Davis, Karen. *National Health Insurance: Benefits, Costs, and Consequences*. Washington, D.C.: The Brookings Institution, 1975.

Derthick, Martha. *The Influence of Federal Grants*. Cambridge, Mass.: Harvard University Press, 1970.

Derthick, Martha. *New Towns In-Town*. Washington, D.C.: The Urban Institute, 1970.

Downs, Anthony. *Inside Bureaucracy*. Boston: Little, Brown, 1967.

Donabedian, Avedis. *A Guide to Medical Care Administration*. Vol. 2. New York: American Public Health Association, 1969.

Ehrenreich, Barbara, and Ehrenreich, John. *The American Health Empire: Power, Profits and Politics*. New York: Vintage Books, 1971.

Feldstein, Martin S. *The Rising Cost of Hospital Care*. Published for National Center for Health Services Research and Development, United States Department of Health, Education, and Welfare. Washington, D.C.: Information Resources Press, 1971.

Georgopolous, Basil S., ed. *Organization Research on Health Institutions*. Ann Arbor: Institute for Social Reserach, University of Michigan, 1972.

Glaser, William A. *Paying the Doctor: Systems of Remuneration and Their Effects*. Baltimore and London: Johns Hopkins Press, 1970.

Harris, Richard. *A Sacred Trust*. Baltimore, Maryland: Penguin Books, Pelican Books, 1969.

Havighurst, Clark C., ed. *Regulating Health Facilities Construction: Proceedings of a Conference on Health Planning, Certificates of Need, and Market Entry*. Washington, D.C.: American Enterprise Institute for Public Policy Research, 1974.

Hoyt, Edwin P. *Condition Critical: Our Hospital Crisis*. New York: Holt, Rinehart, and Winston, 1966.

Kaitz, Edward M. *Pricing Policy and Cost Behavior in the Hospital Industry*. Praeger Special Studies in U.S. Economic and Social Development. New York: Frederick A. Praeger, 1968.

Kaufman, Herbert. *The Limits of Organizational Change*. University, Ala.: University of Alabama Press, 1971.

Kennedy, Senator Edward M. *In Critical Condition: The Crisis in America's Health Care*. New York: Simon and Schuster, 1972.

Lave, Judith R., and Lave, Lester B. *The Hospital Construction Act: An Evaluation of the Hill-Burton Program, 1948-1973*. Evaluative Studies, no. 16. Washington, D.C.: American Enterprise Institute for Public Policy Research, 1974.

Law, Sylvia A., et. al. *Blue Cross: What Went Wrong?* Prepared by the Health Law Project, University of Pennsylvania. New Haven: Yale University Press, 1974.

Levitan, Sar A., ed. *The Federal Social Dollar in Its Own Back Yard*. Washington, D.C.: The Bureau of National Affairs, Inc., 1973.

Marmor, Theodore R., with Jan S. Marmor. *The Politics of Medicare*. 2d ed. Chicago: Aldine Publishing Company, 1973.

Myers, Robert J. *Medicare*. Published for McCahon Foundation, Bryn Mawr, Pennsylvania. Homewood, Illinois: Richard D. Irwin, Inc., 1970.

Noll, Rogert G. *Reforming Regulation: An Evaluation of the Ash Council Proposals*. Studies in the Regulation of Economic Activity. Washington, D.C.: The Brookings Institution, 1971.

O'Donoghue, Patrick. *Evidence about the Effects of Health Care Regulation*. Denver: Spectrum Research, Inc. 1974.

Pauly, Mark V. *Medical Care at Public Expense: A Study in Applied Welfare Economics*. New York: Praeger Publishers, 1971.

Peckman, Joseph A.; Aaron, Henry J.; and Taussig, Michael K. *Social Security: Perspectives for Reform*. Washington, D.C.: The Brookings Institution, 1968.

Pressman, Jeffrey, C., and Wildavsky, Aaron. *Implementation*. Berkeley and Los Angeles: University of California Press, 1973.

Ribicoff, Senator Abraham, with Paul Danaceau. *The American Medical Machine*. New York: Saturday Review Press, 1972.

Schultze, Charles L. with Hamilton, Edward K., and Schick, Allen. *Setting National Priorities: The 1971 Budget*. Washington, D.C.: The Brookings Institution, 1970.

Schwartz, Jerome L. *Medical Plans and Health Care: Consumer Participation in Policy Making with a Special Section on Medicare*. Springfield, Ill.: Charles C. Thomas, 1968.

Sindler, Allan P., ed. *Policy and Politics in America*. Boston: Little, Brown, 1973.

Skidmore, Max J. *Medicare and the American Rhetoric of Reconciliation*. University, Ala.: University of Alabama Press, 1970.

Somers, Anne R. *Health Care in Transition: Directions for the Future*. Chicago: Hospital Research and Education Trust, 1971.

Somers, Anne R. *Hospital Regulation: The Dilemma of Public Policy*. Research Report no. 112, Industrial Relations Section, Princeton University. Princeton, N.J.: Princeton University Press, 1969.

Somers, Herman M., and Somers, Anne R. *Medicare and the Hospitals: Issues and Prospects*. Washington, D.C.: The Brookings Institution, 1967.

Steiner, Gilbert Y. *Social Insecurity: The Politics of Welfare*. Chicago: Rand McNally and Co., 1966.

Strickland, Stephen P. *U.S. Health Care: What's Wrong and What's Right*. Potomac Associates Book. New York: Universe Books, 1972.

Articles, Papers and Reports

Alford, Robert. "The Political Economy of Health Care: Dynamics Without Change." *Politics and Society* 2 (1972): 127-164.

Ball, Robert M. "Social Security Amendments of 1972: Summary and Legislative History." *Social Security Bulletin* 36(March 1973): 3-25.

Bauer, Katherine G., and Densen, Paul M. "Some Issues in the Incentive Reimbursement Approach to Cost Containment: An Overview." Health Care Policy Discussion Paper no. 7, May 1973. Harvard Center for Community Health and Medical Care Program on Health Care Policy. Harvard University, Boston, Massachusetts.

Cashman, John W.; Bierman, Pearl; and Myers, Beverlee A. "The Why of the Medicare Conditions of Participation." Adapted from talk given by Pearl Bierman at the Federal Bar Association Briefing Conference on Medicare, Washington, D.C., April 20, 1967. Typewritten.

Cashman, John W., and Myers, Beverlee A. "Medicare: Standards of Service in a New Program—Licensure, Certification, Accreditation." *American Journal of Public Health* 57 (July 1967): 1107-17.

Cohen, Wilbur J., and Ball, Robert M. "Social Security Amendments of 1967: Summary and Legislative History." *Social Security Bulletin* 31 (February 1968): 3-19.

Corbin, Mildred, and Krute, Aaron. "Some Aspects of Medicare Experience with Group Practice Prepayment Plans." *Social Security Bulletin* 38 (March 1975): 3-11.

Davis, Karen. "Equal Treatment and Unequal Benefits: The Medicare Program." Paper prepared at The Brookings Institution, November 1973. Xeroxed.

Davis, Karen. "Hospital Costs and the Medicare Program." *Social Security Bulletin* 36 (August 1973): 18-36.

Davis, Karen, and Reynolds, Roger. "Medicare and the Utilization of Health Services by the Elderly." Paper prepared at the Brookings Institution, December 1973. Xeroxed.

Davis, Karen. "Theories of Hospital Inflation: Some Empirical Evidence." *Journal of Human Resources* 8 (Spring 1973): 181-201.

Feldstein, Martin. "Welfare Loss of Excess Health Insurance." *Journal of Political Economy* 81 (March-April 1973): 251-80.

Ginsburg, Paul B. "Resource Allocation in the Hospital Industry: The Role of Capital Financing." *Social Security Bulletin* 35 (October 1972): 20-30.

Glaser, William A. " 'Socialized Medicine' in Practice." *The Public Interest.* Spring 1966, pp. 90-106.

Hair, Feather Davis. "Hospital Accreditation: A Developmental Study of the Social Control of Institutions." Ph.D. dissertation, Vanderbilt University, 1972.

Havighurst, Clark C. "Health Maintenance Organizations and the Market for Health Services." *Law and Contemporary Problems* 35 (1970): 716-95.

Havighurst, Clark C. "Regulation of Health Facilities and Service by 'Certificate of Need'." *Virginia Law Review* 59 (1973): 1143-1232.

Horowitz, Loucele A. "Medical Care Price Changes Under the Economic Stabilization Program." Reprinted from the *Social Security Bulletin,* June 1973. U.S., Department of Health, Education, and Welfare, Social Security Administration. DHEW Publication no. (SSA) 73-11700.

Iglehart, John K. "Explosive Rise in Medical Costs Puts Government in Quandary." *National Journal* 7 (1975): 1319-28.

Iglehart, John K. "Health Report/Democrats Cool to Nixon's Health Proposal, Offer their own Alternatives." *National Journal* 3 (1971): 2310ff.

Iglehart, John K. "Health Report/Prepaid Group Medicare Practice Emerges as Likely Federal Approach to Health Care." *National Journal* 3 (1971): 1443-52.

Jones, Ellen W.; Densen, Paul M.; Altman, Isidore; Shapiro, Sam; and West, Howard. "HIP Incentive Reimbursement Experiment: Utilization and Costs of Medical Care 1969 and 1970." *Social Security Bulletin* 37 (December 1974): 3-34.

Kirsch, Lawrence J. "An Analysis of the Proposed Hill-Burton Regulations Governing Medical Services for Persons Unable to Pay." Health Care Policy Discussion Paper no. 1, June 1972. Harvard Center for Community Health and Medical Care, Program on Health Care Policy. Harvard University, Boston, Massachusetts.

Lazin, Frederick Aaron. "The Failure of Federal Enforcement of Civil Rights Regulations in Public Housing, 1963-1971: The Cooptation of a Federal Agency by Its Local Constituency." *Policy Sciences* 4(1973): 263-73.

Lindblom, Charles E. "The Science of Muddling Through." *Public Administration Review* 19 (1959): 79-88.

Marmor, T., and Thomas, D. "The Politics of Paying Physicians: The Determinants of Government Payment Methods in England, Sweden, and the United States." *International Journal of Health Services* 1 (1971): 21-78.

Murphy, Jerome T. "Title I of ESEA: The Politics of Implementing Federal Education Reform." *Harvard Educational Review* 41 (February 1971): 35-63.

National Academy of Public Administration. "Final Report on the Medicare Project Panel." Submitted to Arthur Hess, Acting Commissioner of Social Security, June 30, 1973.

Newman, H.F. "Medicare and the Comprehensive Health Cooperative of Puget Sound." *Bulletin of the New York Academy of Medicine* 44 (November 1968): 1312-20.

Newman, H.F. "The Impact of Medicare on Group Practice Prepayment Plans." *American Journal of Public Health* 59 (April 1969): 619-24.

Note. "The Role of Prepaid Group Practice in Relieving the Medical Care Crisis." *Harvard Law Review* 84 (February 1971): 887-1001.

Pauly, M. and Redisch, M. "The Not-for-Profit Hospital as a Physician's Cooperative." *American Economic Review* 63 (March 1973): 87-99.

Posner, Richard. "Taxation by Regulation." *Bell Journal of Economics and Management Science* 2 (1971): 22-50.

Rowland, Diane. "Data Rich and Information Poor: Medicare's Resources for Prospective Rate-Setting." Harvard University Center for Community Health and Medical Care, Report Series R-45-12, July 1976.

Smith, Bruce L. R., and Hollander, Neil, eds. "The Administration of Medicare: A Shared Responsibility." Papers prepared for the Belmont Conference on the Administration of Medicare, September 27-28, 1972. Washington, D.C.: National Academy of Public Administration, 1973.

Tierney, Thomas M. "Medicare and the Financing of Teaching Hospitals." *Journal of Medical Education* 44 (1969): 907-11.

West, Howard. "Group Practice Prepayment Plans in the Medicare Program," *American Journal of Public Health* 59 (April 1969): 624-29.

Wilson, James Q. "The Politics of American Business Regulation." In *Social Responsibility: A Business Predicament*, edited by James McKie. Washington, D.C.: The Brookings Institution, 1974.

Wolkstein, Irwin. "Comprehensive Health Planning and Financing." Presented before American Hospital Association Institute on Capital Financing for Hospitals, Chicago, April 1, 1969. Xeroxed.

Wolkstein, Irwin. "Incentive Reimbursement and Group Practice Prepayment." In *Proceedings*. 19th Annual Group Health Institute, June 4-6, 1969. Washington, D.C.: Group Health Association of America, 1969.

Wolkstein, Irwin. "Incentive Reimbursement Plans Offer a Wide Variety of Approaches to Cost Control." *Hospitals* 43(1969): 63-67.

Wolkstein, Irwin. "Overview of Budget Review Systems of Reimbursement." *Hospital Forum* (December 1972): 11–14.

Wolkstein, Irwin. "Prospective Rate Setting–The Engineer's Role in Cost Finding or Justification." Presented before American Hospital Association Institute on Hospital Management Systems, Denver, Colorado, February 1, 1971. Xeroxed.

Wolkstein, Irwin. "Public Policy in Reimbursement." Presented at 1969 Health Administrators Development Program, Cornell University, July 11, 1969. Xeroxed.

Wolkstein, Irwin. "The American Hospital Association Statement on Financial Requirements and Some Comparisons with Medicare Reimbursement." Presented before the Third Annual Institute of the Northeast Ohio Chapter, Hospital Financial Management Association, Cleveland, Ohio, October 23, 1969. Xeroxed.

Worthington, William, and Silver, Laurens H. "Regulation of Quality of Care in Hospitals: The Need for Change." In "Health Care: Part I". *Law and Contemporary Problems* 35:2 (Spring 1970) pp. 305–33. Published by the Duke University School of Law, Durham, N.C., copyright 1970, 1971 by Duke University.

For consumer-oriented articles on Medicare and health policy in general, see articles by Mal Schecter, Washington Editor, *Hospital Practice*.

For reports on ongoing federal policy on Medicare and the health care field, see "Washington Report on Medicine and Health." Washington, D.C.: McGraw-Hill.

Government Documents

U.S., Congress, House, Committee on Government Operations. *Administration of Federal Health Benefits Programs: Hearings before Subcommittee.* 91st Cong., 2d sess., 1970; and 92d Cong., 1st and 2d sess., 1972.

U.S., Congress, House, Committee on Interstate and Foreign Commerce, Subcommittee on Public Health and Welfare. *Hospital and Health Facility Construction and Modernization: Hearings.* 91st Cong., 1st sess., 1969.

U.S., Congress, House, Committee on Ways and Means. *Medical Care for the Aged: Executive Hearings before the Committee on Ways and Means on H.R. 1 and other Proposals for Medical Care for the Aged.* 89th Cong., 1st sess., 1965.

_____. *President's Proposals for Revision of the Social Security System: Hearings on H.R. 5710.* 90th Cong., 1st sess., 1967.

_____. *Social Security Amendments of 1970: Report on H.R. 17550.* H.R. 91–1096. 91st Cong., 2d sess., 1970.

_____. *Social Security Amendments of 1971: Report on H.R. 1*. H.R. 92–231. 92d Cong., 1st sess., 1971.

_____. *Social Security and Welfare Proposals: Hearings*. 91st Cong., 1st sess., 1970.

U.S., Congress, Senate, Committee on Finance. *Medicare and Medicaid: Hearings*. 91st Cong., 1st sess., 1969.

_____. *Medicare and Medicaid: Hearings*. Part 1. 91st Cong., 2d sess., 1970.

_____. *Medicare and Medicaid: Hearings*. Part 2. 91st Cong., 2d sess., 1970.

_____. *Medicare and Medicaid: Problems, Issues, and Alternatives; Report of the Staff to the Committee on Finance*. 91st Cong., 1st sess., 1970.

_____. *National Health Insurance: Hearings*. 92d Cong., 1st sess., 1971.

_____. *Reimbursement Guidelines for Medicare: Executive Hearings*. 89th Cong., 2d sess., May 25, 1966.

_____. *Social Security: Hearings on H.R. 6675*. 89th Cong., 1st sess., 1965.

_____. *Social Security Amendments of 1967: Hearings on H.R. 12080*. 90th Cong., 1st sess., 1967.

_____. *Social Security Amendments of 1970: Hearings on H.R. 17550*. 91st Cong., 2d sess., 1970.

_____. *Social Security Amendments of 1971: Hearings on H.R. 1*. 92d Cong., 1st and 2d sess., 1971 and 1972.

_____. *Social Security Amendments of 1970: Report to Accompany H.R. 17550*. S.R. 91–1431. 91st Cong., 2d sess., 1970.

_____. *Social Security Amendments of 1972: Report to Accompany H.R. 1*. S.R. 92–1230. 92d Cong., 2d sess., 1972.

_____. *Social Security Amendments of 1973: Report to Accompany H.R. 3153*. S.R. 93–653. 93d Cong., 1st sess., 1973.

U.S., Congress, Senate, Committee on Government Operations, Subcommittee on Executive Reorganization. *Health Care in America: Hearings*. 90th Cong., 2d sess., 1969.

U.S., Congress, Senate, Committee on the Judiciary, Subcommittee on Antitrust and Monopoly. *High Cost of Hospitalization: Hearings*. 91st Cong., 2d sess., 1970 and 1971.

U.S., Congress, Senate, Committee on Labor and Public Welfare, Subcommittee on Health. *Health Care Crisis in America, 1971: Hearings*. 92d Cong., 1st sess., 1971.

_____. *Medical Care Facilities Construction and Modernization: Hearings*. 91st Cong., 1st sess., 1969.

U.S., Congress, Senate, Special Committee on Aging. *Costs and Delivery of Health Services to Older Americans: Hearings*. 90th Cong., 1st and 2d sess., 1968 and 1969.

U.S., Department of Health, Education and Welfare. *Report of Task Force on Medicaid and Related Programs*. June 1970.

_____. Report on National Conference on Medical Costs (held June 27-28, 1967), 1968. Papers prepared for this conference were made available to me by Susan Jenkins of SSA and should now be available in the SSA library, Baltimore.

_____. Social Security Administration. *Background on Medicare, 1957-1962: Reports, Studies and Congressional Considerations on Health Legislation.* 2 vols., 85th-87th Congress. Available in the library of the Social Security Administration, Baltimore, Maryland.

_____. Social Security Administration, Office of Research and Statistics, *Community Hospitals: Inflation in the Pre-Medicare Period.* Research Report no 4, by Karen Davis and Richard W. Foster. Washington, D.C.: Government Printing Office, 1972.

_____. Social Security Administration, Office of Research and Statistics. *The Evolution of Medicare . . . from Idea to Law.* Research Report no. 29, by Peter A. Corning. Washington, D.C.: Government Printing Office, 1969.

_____. Social Security Administration, Office of Research and Statistics. *Net Income of Hospitals, 1961-69.* Staff Paper no. 6 by Karen Davis. December 1970.

_____. Social Security Administration, Office of Research and Statistics. *Reimbursement Incentives for Hospital and Medical Care: Objectives and Alternatives.* Research Report no. 26. Washington, D.C.: Government Printing Office, 1968.

U.S., Economic Stabilization Program, Cost of Living Council. "Phase II and Phase III Controls on the Hospital Sector." Prepared for the Staff of the Health Advisory Committee and the Cost of Living Council Committee on Health by Robert E. Schlenker and Richard McNeil, Jr. April 1973. Xeroxed.

U.S., General Accounting Office, Comptroller General. *Additional Information on Certain Aspects of Independent and Hospital-Based Laboratories.* B-164031 (4). August 1, 1973.

_____. Report to the Chairman, Committee on Finance, U.S. Senate, by the Comptroller General. *Evaluation of Department of Health, Education, and Welfare Proposed Regulation Changes Affecting Medicare Reimbursement to Institutions.* B-164031 (4). March 24, 1972.

_____. Report to the Committee on Finance, U.S. Senate, by the Comptroller General. *Better Controls Needed for Health Maintenance Organizations Under Medicaid in California.* B-164031 (3). Social and Rehabilitation Service, Department of Health, Education, and Welfare, September 10, 1974.

_____. Report to the Committee on Finance, U.S. Senate, by the Comptroller General. *Medicare Payments for Services of Supervisory and Teaching Physicians at Cook County Hospital, Chicago, Illinois.* B-164031 (4). Social Security Administration, Department of Health, Education, and Welfare. September 3, 1969.

————. Report to the Committee on Finance, U.S. Senate, by the Comptroller General. *Payments to Hospitals and Extended Care Facilities for Depreciation Expense Under the Medicare Program*. B-142983. Social Security Administration, Department of Health, Education, and Welfare. August 21, 1970.

————. Report to the Committee on the Judiciary, House of Representatives, by the Comptroller General. *Compliance with the Antidiscrimination Provision of Civil Rights Act by Hospitals and Other Facilities Under Medicare and Medicaid*. B-164031 (4). Department of Health, Education, and Welfare. July 13, 1972.

————. Report to the Congress by the Comptroller General. *Improved Controls Needed Over Extent of Care Provided by Hospitals and Other Facilities to Medicare Patients*. B-164031 (4). Social Security Administration, Department of Health, Education, and Welfare. July 30, 1971.

————. Report to the Congress by the Comptroller General. *Lengthy Delays in Settling the Costs of Health Services Furnished Under Medicare*. B-164031 (4). Social Security Administration, Department of Health, Education, and Welfare. July 23, 1971.

————. Report to the Congress by the Comptroller General. *Need for Legislation to Authorize More Economical Ways of Providing Durable Medical Equipment Under Medicare*. B-164031 (4). Social Security Administration, Department of Health, Education, and Welfare. May 12, 1972.

————. Report to the Congress by the Comptroller General. *Need for Timely Action in Resolving Problems Affecting the Eligibility of Hospitals Under the Medicare Program*. B-164031 (4). Social Security Administration, Department of Health, Education, and Welfare. December 27, 1968.

————. Report to the Congress by the Comptroller General. *Problems Associated with Reimbursement to Hospitals for Services Furnished Under Medicare*. B-164031 (4). Social Security Administration, Department of Health, Education, and Welfare. August 3, 1972.

————. Report to the Congress by the Comptroller General. *Problems in Paying for Services of Supervisory and Teaching Physicians in Hospitals Under Medicare*. B-164031 (4). Social Security Administration, Department of Health, Education, and Welfare. November 17, 1971.

————. Report to the Congress by the Comptroller General. *Sizable Amounts Due the Government by Institutions that Terminated Their Participation in the Medicare Program*. B-164031 (4). Social Security Administration, Department of Health, Education, and Welfare. August 4, 1972.

————. Report to the Congress by the Comptroller General. *Study of Health Facilities Construction Costs*. B-164031 (3). November 20, 1972.

————. Report to the Secretary of Health, Education, and Welfare. *Administrative Costs of the Medicare Program Can Be Reduced by Authorizing*

Contractors to Use Government Sources of Supply. B-164031 (4). Social Security Administration, Department of Health, Education, and Welfare. July 21, 1970.

————. Report to the Secretary of Health, Education, and Welfare by the Comptroller General. *Problems in Determining the Reasonableness of Physicians' Charges Under the Medicare Program in Massachusetts*. B-164031 (4). Social Security Administration, Department of Health, Education, and Welfare. June 30, 1969.

————. Statement of George J. Ahart, Director, Manpower and Welfare Division, before Subcommittee no. 4, Committee on the Judiciary, U.S. House of Representatives, on Compliance with Antidiscrimination Provision of Civil Rights Act by Hospitals and Other Facilities Under Medicare and Medicaid. September 12, 1973. Xeroxed.

U.S., President of the U.S., National Advisory Commission on Health Facilities. *Report to the President*. December 1968.

U.S., President of the U.S. *Report of the National Advisory Commission on Health Manpower*, 2 vols. 1967 and 1968.

U.S., Secretary of Health, Education, and Welfare. *Report of the 1971 Advisory Council on Social Security*. House Document No. 92-80. 92d Cong., 1st sess., 1971.

Much of the material on policy considerations between 1965 and 1971 comes from the minutes and staff papers of the Health Insurance Benefits Advisory Council. I am indebted to Kermit Gordon and Charles Schultze, the first two chairmen of the council, for use of their copies of these documents.

Index

Eligibility, hospital. *See also* Certification
for Medicare program, 4, 5
Emergency Maternity and Infant Care
Program, 53
Enforcement, of JCAH standards, 8
balancing strategy for, 45
via claims denial, 41
objections to, 21
SSA decision making on, 24
Executive. *See also* Nixon administration
and Medicare policy, 156
Expansion, hospital. *See also* Construction
vs. costs, 59
Expenditures, hospital. *See also* Costs
increases in, 81
Experimentations proposals. *See also*
Group Practice Prepayment
Plans
attitudes toward, 91
for HMOs, 133
Extended care facilities (ECFs), 41,
116
assurance of payment procedure
for, 50n
certification of, 22
medicare payments for, 123

Federal agencies. *See also* Governmental agencies; *specific
agencies*
compromise policies of, 150
Federal budget, and rising hospital
costs, 111
Federal health programs, Medicare
and, 40
Fee-for-service system
cost-effective medical organizations
in, 131
and hospital profit, 114
Finance Committee, Senate, 23, 34,
36, 37, 41, 44, 67, 100
on accelerated depreciation, 123
allocation options advocated by,
125

on cost containment, 155
on cost limits, 121
on HMOs, 131
initial reimbursement regulations
and, 88
investigation of Medicare administration, 117–119
on reimbursement capital, 69
Fiscal agents, appointed by BHI, 86,
109
"Fiscal intermediary." *See also* Intermediaries
concept of, 37
Florida, hospital certification in, 18
Fountain, Congressman, 98, 100

Gardner, J., 65
General Accounting Office (GAO), 96
on accelerated depreciation, 124
certification evaluation by, 16–17
investigations of, 129
Glasser, M., 38
Gordon, K., 59
Gorham Report, 92
Government agencies. *See also* Federal agencies; State agencies
policy goals of, 150
Government Operations Committee,
House, 97, 98, 125
Group Health Association of America
(GHAA), 84
Group Health Cooperative, of Puget
Sound, 133, 141n
Group Practice Prepayment Plans
(GPPPs)
Group Health Cooperative of Puget
Sound, 133, 141n
lobbyists for, 132
payment of, 82–87
reimbursement experimentation
with, 91
test of medical care management
under, 107n
Growth, hospital. *See also* Construction
Medicare financing of, 54
Guidelines, for hospital certification,15

About the Author

Judith M. Feder is a research associate at The Urban Institute, Washington, D.C., where she is continuing health policy research. She completed this book as a service fellow at the National Center for Health Services Research, Department of Health, Education and Welfare. Prior to her appointment there, she was a senior health policy analyst at the Government Research Corporation, Washington, D.C. Ms. Feder received the Ph.D. in political science from Harvard University and is specializing in the politics of health.